Hanane Boukrous

Potential New Biomarkers Of Diabetic Nephropathy 2

Hanane Boukrous

Potential New Biomarkers Of Diabetic Nephropathy 2

ScienciaScripts

Imprint

Cover image: www.ingimage.com

This book is a translation from the original published under ISBN 978-620-6-71058-5.

Publisher:
Sciencia Scripts
is a trademark of
Dodo Books Indian Ocean Ltd. and OmniScriptum S.R.L publishing group

120 High Road, East Finchley, London, N2 9ED, United Kingdom
Str. Armeneasca 28/1, office 1, Chisinau MD-2012, Republic of Moldova, Europe
Managing Directors: Ieva Konstantinova, Victoria Ursu
info@omniscriptum.com

Printed at: see last page
ISBN: 978-620-8-38502-6

Contents

Introduction

Diabetes mellitus (DM) is a complex disease. The wealth of data on new technologies and treatments is rapidly advancing our knowledge of diabetes and its complications and our ability to manage them, but poses challenges for doctors and other healthcare professionals (1) . It also places a heavy economic burden on sufferers and their families, as well as on national healthcare systems (2).

The pathophysiology behind this complex and heterogeneous disease distinguishes between different types of diabetes: type 1 diabetes (T1DM), type 2 diabetes (T2DM) and gestational diabetes (3).

It has been suggested that T1DM and T2DM represent the extremes of the diabetic disease spectrum and that the traditional dichotomous classification is giving way to an increasingly nuanced classification (4).

Unfortunately, T2DM has become a real public health problem, not only because of its high and steadily rising prevalence, which accounts for almost 90% of cases, but also because of the associated pathologies, in particular cardiovascular disease, which is responsible for a high morbidity and mortality rate (5).

In fact, the prevalence of T2DM increases sharply with age "the age of onset of the disease has shifted towards young adults and even adolescents over the last few decades" due to the development of obesity, a sedentary lifestyle and excessive energy intake (5).

The complications attributable to this pandemic are numerous, local or general, insidious, chronic and often serious, since the life span of a diabetic is shortened by five to ten years (6).

The great classics - the result of the combined deleterious effects of microangiopathy and macroangiopathy, which are linked by similar mechanisms - remain, but their presentation has changed with the improvement in therapeutic management, the emergence of new concepts and the ageing of the diabetic population (6).

Diabetic nephropathy (DN) is one of the most serious microvascular complications of diabetes (6), which has become the leading cause of end-stage renal disease (ESRD). Nephropathy is primarily the consequence of microangiopathy. Today, T2DM is the leading cause of admission to dialysis in Europe.

The mechanisms of renal failure in T2DM are complex, interlinked and often uncertain, since a renal biopsy is only performed in 20% of cases (and is rarely used because it is invasive and there are no strict clinical indications at this stage of the disease). It is very difficult to distinguish between a genuine complication of diabetes and a comorbidity associated with diabetes. In addition to microangiopathy, which is mainly linked to the effect of hyperglycaemia on glomerular morphology and function, there are the adverse effects of age, arterial hypertension (AH) and atherosclerosis, to such an extent that progression to renal failure also marks a stage in the progression of cardiovascular risk (6).

The stereotypical history of diabetic nephropathy begins with an increase in urinary albumin excretion (microalbuminuria), the initial sign of glomerular damage,

progressing at a rate of 2.8% per year towards macro-proteinemia and then, at an annual rate of 2.3%, towards renal failure, according to data from the UKPDS (UK prospective diabetic study) (6).
These different stages are accompanied by histological lesions that remain silent for a long time, progressing from the stage of glomerular hypertrophy to thickening of the glomerular basement membrane, followed by mesangial expansion and accumulation of extracellular matrix in the glomerulus.
This sequence, which is well described in T1DM, is much more difficult to identify in T2DM, where macroangiopathy undermines the disease both synchronously and independently.
It is therefore essential to identify any deterioration in renal function at an early stage by measuring creatinine (to estimate glomerular filtration rate) and microalbuminuria annually (6).
However, these investigative tools have had their limitations in use and are sometimes insensitive to the detection of early renal failure.
Indeed, it has been found that urinary albumin excretion (UAE) and decline in glomerular filtration rate (GFR) can occur separately and in a complementary fashion: normo albuminuric nephropathy. This implies that albuminuria is unable to predict ND and progression to ESRD in all patients and raises important questions as to whether these two markers of renal dysfunction differ in terms of pathogenic mechanisms, prognostic implications and therapeutic measures (7).
Microalbuminuria, which is an important "gold standard" indicator for assessing the progression of diabetic nephropathy, in particular with a decline in glomerular filtration rate, is not precise enough to assess severity or prognosis simply on the basis of the degree of proteinuria. All the more so since, according to the natural history of the development of ND established by Mogensen in the late 1980s (8), urinary albumin excretion (UAE), which appears five or even more years after diabetes has progressed for ten years, microalbuminuria is not seen until stage three of the progression of ND. So the disease is clinically silent until an advanced stage.
In the absence of detection and intervention, patients run the risk of suffering significant irreversible damage or dying as a result of their kidney failure. Earlier detection will not only contribute to the clinical management of patients, but will also stimulate research into new therapies for kidney disease (9).
In addition, impaired renal function may be present even in patients with normal urinary albumin excretion. This suggests the need to screen patients several years before the onset of microalbuminuria (8).
On the other hand, GFR, whose estimation is based on a simple endogenous biomarker, is poorly assessed by determining serum creatinine alone (which depends on muscle mass, meat consumption and age) (10).
A great deal of effort has gone into developing an accurate estimate of glomerular filtration rate, which is why several equations incorporating anthropometric data have been used to estimate GFR. The most widely used and recommended are the simple

but not very accurate Cockcroft-Gault formula. To compensate for this, other more recent equations (Modification of Diet in Renal Disease (MDRD) Mayo Clinic Quadratic, CKD-EPI) have been established on the basis of populations including subjects without renal failure (11).

However, the best procedures for estimating glomerular filtration rate depend on the elimination of 51Cr- EDTA or iohexol, which are rarely used in clinical settings or for large-scale research studies (11) .

To overcome all these controversies, it would make sense to measure biomarkers of renal function that could optimise strategies for the early detection, prevention and treatment of diabetic nephropathy.

In order to correctly qualify the potential markers of renal damage in T2DM, it is useful to classify them according to the renal structure affected by the pathological process.

On this basis, a distinction is made between markers of glomerular damage including transferrin, immunoglobulin G (IgG), ceruleoplasmin, cystatin C (Cys C) and nephrin, and markers of tubular damage such as neutrophil lipocalin associated with gelatinase (NGAL), alpha-1-microglobulin; kidney injury molecule-1 (KIM-1) and beta 2 microglobulin (ß2-M) (12).

Cys-C has been proposed as an alternative endogenous serum biomarker for the estimation of renal function. Cys C is a protein that is freely filtered in the glomerulus and almost entirely reabsorbed and catabolised by the epithelial cells of the proximal tubules. Its synthesis is thought to be constant and unaffected by muscle mass or diet, age or inflammatory conditions (13).

Like ß2-M, which is a key component of the adaptive immune system, it is also freely filtered in the glomerulus, then completely reabsorbed and metabolised by the epithelial cells of the proximal tubules. Its levels increase when renal function declines (14).

It is therefore essential to always identify a simple, reliable, unambiguous and reproducible marker to detect kidney damage at an early stage.

Despite this plethora of knowledge, the scientific community is only just beginning to convert the screening of these biomarkers into standard clinical practice in order to offer patients appropriate treatment. A technique based on urinary proteomics, known as the chronic kidney disease 273(*CKD*) classifier, has been developed to predict the progression of CKD and distinguish CKD patients according to disease severity. Extending this proteomic screening to include indicators of oxidative stress and inflammation and tubular biomarkers, as well as a metabolomic approach, could further improve prognosis (15).

The challenge remains great, but knowledge of kidney disease in the context of diabetes is improving. We can therefore expect progress in the near future to reduce this defect, which degrades patients' quality of life, jeopardises their vitality and adds considerably to healthcare costs (16).

CHAPTER 1

2.1. Diabetes mellitus

2.1.1. Definition and diagnostic criteria

2.1.1.1. Definition

DM is a group of metabolic diseases characterised by chronic hyperglycaemia that occurs when the pancreas does not produce insulin, or does not produce enough insulin, or when the body is unable to use the insulin it produces correctly (3, 17).

Diabetes is a major public health problem, and is one of the four priority non-communicable diseases targeted by world leaders. A steady increase in the number of cases of diabetes and in the prevalence of the disease has been recorded in recent decades (18).

2.1.1.2. Diagnostic criteria

The diagnosis of diabetes can be made in three different ways, which, in the absence of obvious hyperglycaemia, will need to be confirmed by a second measurement:

- Symptoms of diabetes (polyuria, polydipsia, unexplained weight loss, drowsiness or even coma) and blood glucose at any time >2.00 g/L (11.1 mmol/L). -Fasting blood glucose >1.26 g/L (7.00 mmol/L).
- Blood glucose 2 h after a 75 g glucose load in hyperglycaemia oral glucose tolerance (OGTT) >2.00 g/L (11.1 mmol/L).

The International Expert Committee on Diabetes, set up in 1995 at the request of the ADA, has proposed a new categorisation and diagnostic criteria for diabetes (17).

In 2010, the ADA approved the use of glycated haemoglobin (HbA1c) as a diagnostic biomarker for diabetes and pre-diabetes based on the recommendations of a panel of international experts including representatives from the ADA, the International Diabetes Federation (IDF) and the European Association for the Diabetes Study (EADS). The Swiss Society of Endocrinology recently approved the application of these recommendations in Switzerland (19).

Table 1: criteria for diagnosing diabetes (20)

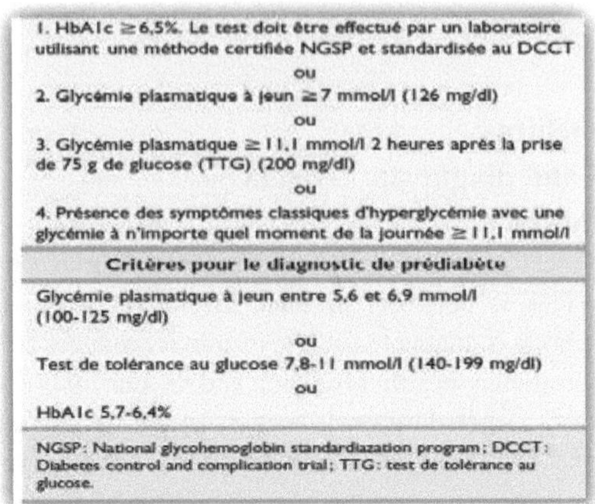

1. HbA1c ≥6,5%. Le test doit être effectué par un laboratoire utilisant une méthode certifiée NGSP et standardisée au DCCT

ou

2. Glycémie plasmatique à jeun ≥7 mmol/l (126 mg/dl)

ou

3. Glycémie plasmatique ≥11,1 mmol/l 2 heures après la prise de 75 g de glucose (TTG) (200 mg/dl)

ou

4. Présence des symptômes classiques d'hyperglycémie avec une glycémie à n'importe quel moment de la journée ≥11,1 mmol/l

Critères pour le diagnostic de prédiabète

Glycémie plasmatique à jeun entre 5,6 et 6,9 mmol/l (100-125 mg/dl)

ou

Test de tolérance au glucose 7,8-11 mmol/l (140-199 mg/dl)

ou

HbA1c 5,7-6,4%

NGSP: National glycohemoglobin standardiazation program; DCCT: Diabetes control and complication trial; TTG: test de tolérance au glucose.

For the World Health Organisation (WHO), an HbA1c level > 6.5% is a diagnostic criterion for diabetes, but not for intermediate hyperglycaemia, because the quality of assurance of HbA1c measurement is not available worldwide. Currently, the WHO recommends a two-hour OGTT to detect impaired glucose tolerance and impaired fasting glucose. However, a growing body of reliable evidence suggests that a one-hour OGTT is a more reasonable method for detecting intermediate hyperglycaemia at any given time (18).

2.1.2.Classification

In 1965, the WHO published its first report on the classification of diabetes, which was based on one major criterion, age; four age groups were covered in this report (21).

Updates were adopted in 1980 and 1985 respectively; these classification reports included two types of diabetes: insulin-dependent diabetes mellitus, sometimes known as type 1 diabetes (T1DM), and non-insulin-dependent type 2; in addition, they introduced two other classes of DM: "other types of diabetes" and gestational diabetes. However, the 1985 report omitted the terms "T1DM" and "T2DM", and introduced the class of DM related to relativistic malnutrition diabetes mellitus (DMDM) (21).

These categories were included in the International Classification of Diseases in 1991, and in the tenth revision of the International Classification of Diseases in 1992. The nosological classification of diabetes published in 1997 by a group of experts under the responsibility of the ADA replaces that drawn up in 1979 by the National Diabetes Data group and endorsed in 1980 by the WHO (22).

The WHO proposed in 1999 that categorisation should encompass not only the many aetiologies of diabetes, but also the different clinical phases of the disease. It therefore reintroduced the terms T1DM and T2DM but at the same time removed the notion of DMDM due to the lack of evidence to support its existence as a distinct type (21).

Ideally, a single classification system for diabetes would meet three main objectives: clinical care, aetiopathology and epidemiology. With this in mind, leading learned societies have considered that the ideal is to define a classification system that prioritises clinical care and helps healthcare professionals choose appropriate treatments and decide whether or not to start insulin therapy (21).

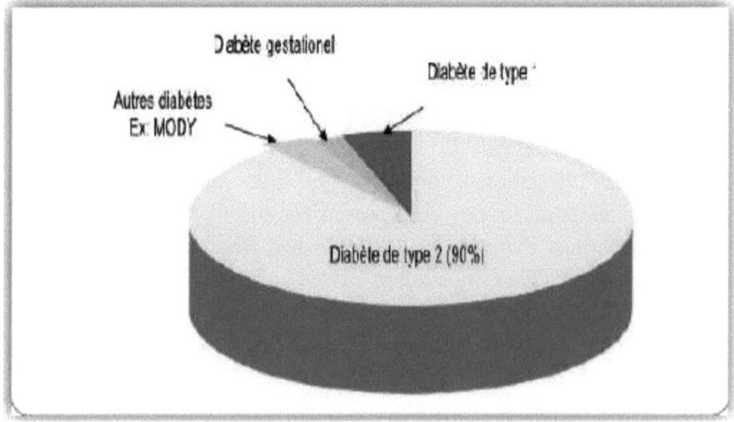

Figure 1: WHO classification of diabetes (4)

The only classification system that could currently do this is one based on clinical parameters to identify diabetes subtypes. Such a classification based on these measures would have limited global applicability (21).

1.1.1.1. Type 1 diabetes

It accounts for less than 10% of diabetes cases. It corresponds to the destruction of the Langerhans beta cell, usually resulting in absolute insulin deficiency. It is divided into 2 subtypes:

> Autoimmune T1DM

During which the destruction of beta cells by an autoimmune process is authenticated by the presence of anti-islet cell, anti-insulin, anti-glutamate decarboxylase and anti-tyrosine phosphatase antibodies. Autoimmune diabetes can occur at any age, including after the age of 70 (21).

^ Idiopathic T1DM

Affects a minority of patients. Some present with permanent insulinopenia with ketoacidosis of unknown origin; this form, which has a strong hereditary component, is more frequent in subjects of African or Asian origin. In Africans, a similar form is characterised by a revealing ketoacidosis after which insulin therapy is not essential (17) .

T1DM is one of the most common chronic diseases of childhood, although T2DM also occurs in older children and is on the increase due to the greater prevalence of overweight and obesity in children (2).

1.1.1.2. Type 2 diabetes

T2DM is the most common type, accounting for around 90% of all cases of diabetes worldwide (2).

T2DM corresponds to the old terminology of non-insulin-dependent DM and associates dominant insulin resistance with relative insulinopenia, a predominant reduction in insulin secretion associated or not with insulin resistance (21).

1.1.1.3. Gestational diabetes

Gestational diabetes is one of the most frequent complications of pregnancy, with a prevalence ranging from 1 to 25%, depending on the country, ethnic group, age and body mass index (BMI) (23).

The WHO defines gestational diabetes as glucose intolerance leading to hyperglycaemia of variable severity, diagnosed for the first time during pregnancy. Gestational diabetes must therefore be distinguished from a pregnancy in a woman with previously known diabetes, most often T1DM but also T2DM or MODY (23).

The main complications associated with gestational diabetes are macrosomia (with a prevalence of 15-30%), gestational hypertension and pre-eclampsia, and the risk of the woman developing T2DM in the years following delivery (24).

1.1.1.4. Other types of diabetes

Single gene diabetes, as its name suggests, results from the mutation of a single gene. It is much less common, accounting for 1.5 to 2% of all cases, although these figures may be underestimated: it is often misdiagnosed as T1DM or T2DM.

These monogenic forms cover a wide spectrum, from neonatal DM (sometimes called "monogenic childhood diabetes") to maturity-onset diabetes of the young (MODY), including rare syndromic diseases associated with diabetes (2).

A further distinction between the fourteen different subtypes of MODY diabetes leads not only to differences in clinical management but also to different predictions of the risk of complications (2).

Table 2: WHO and ADA classification of diabetes mellitus in 1988 (25)

1. Diabète sucré de type 1
   a. auto-immun (trouble des cellules β)
   b. idiopathique (rare, sans élément pour facteur auto-immun)
2. Diabète sucré de type 2 (résistance à l'insuline et défaut de sécrétion d'insuline)
3. Types spécifiques de diabète
   a. Défaut génétique de la fonction des cellules β (Maturity Diabetes of the Young: MODY). Actuellement, cinq défauts différents sont connus dans le diabète de type MODY:
      MODY 1: défaut de l'Hepatocyte nuclear factor 4α (HNF-4α)
      MODY 2: défaut de la glucosinase
      MODY 3: défaut de l'HNF-1α
      MODY 4: défaut de l'IPT-1 (insulin promoter factor-1)
      MODY 5: défaut de l'HNF-1α, diabète mitochondrial, autres
   b. Défaut génétique dans l'action de l'insuline (résistance à l'insuline de type A, Lepréchaunisme, syndrome de Rabson-Mendenhall: défaut des récepteurs à l'insuline, diabète lipo-atrophique, autres)
   c. Maladies du pancréas exocrine (pancréatite, néoplasie, fibrose kystique, hémochromatose, pancréatopathie fibro-calculeuse, autres)
   d. Endocrinopathies (acromégalie, syndrome de Cushing, phéochromocytome, syndrome de Conn, autres)
   e. Induit par les médicaments (stéroïdes, pentamidine, acide nicotinique, diazoxyde, thiazides, inhibiteurs de la protéase, autres)
   f. Infections (rougeole congénitale, oreillons, virus Coxsackie, cytomégalovirus)
   g. Formes rares de diabète immunogène (syndrome de Stiff-Man, anticorps anti-insuline-récepteurs, autres)
   h. Autres syndromes génétiques associés au diabète (trisomie 21, syndrome de Klinefelter, syndrome de Turner, dystrophie myotonique, autres)
4. Diabète gestationnel

Other pathologies can also cause diabetes: specific types of diabetes according to the most recent WHO classification of diabetes (21) (table 2).

2.1.3. Prevalence of diabetes

2.1.3.1. Prevalence of diabetes worldwide

Demographic growth and the ageing of the population have contributed in 40% of cases to an increase in the number of diabetics: the number of people with diabetes rose significantly between 1980 and 2014, from 108 million to the current figures, which are around four times higher (26). It should be pointed out that the incidence of this disease is on the rise in regions where there is an increase in overweight and obesity, as well as in regions with high incomes.

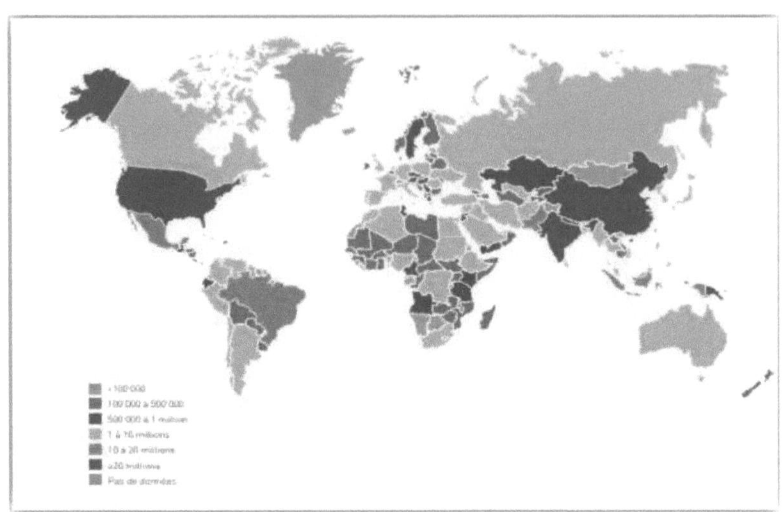

Figure 1: Estimated total number of adults (aged 20 to 79) living with diabetes

in 2019 (2) low and intermediate or diabetes is progressing dramatically (26)Accurate estimates and forecasts of the prevalence of diabetes at global, regional and national levels are necessary for planning and monitoring prevention and treatment strategies (26).

The International Diabetes Federation (IDF) has estimated that worldwide, the prevalence of diabetes in adults aged between 20 and 79 was 8.3% in 2012, which represents 371 million people with diabetes. This number will reach 592 million in 2030 (10.2%) and 700 million in 2045 (10.9%) (27).

2.1.3.2. Prevalence of diabetes in Africa and the Middle East

In Africa, the disease is widespread, although exact figures are rare and controversial; the WHO has reported highly variable frequencies depending on the country. These frequencies are higher in North African countries. In Libya, the prevalence is 9.3%, in Mauritania, for example, the prevalence of diabetes is between 7.2 and 10.5%, 9.9% in Tunisia, 8.7% in Algeria, 7.35% in Morocco and 9.3% in Egypt (27).

The prevalence of diabetes was significantly higher in urban areas (9%) than in rural areas (4.4%). It did not vary significantly between the sexes, either in urban areas (8.8 vs. 9.2%) or in rural areas (4.8 vs. 4.1%). Prevalence increases with age: 2.3% in the 20-34 age group and 13.1% in those aged 65 and over (28).

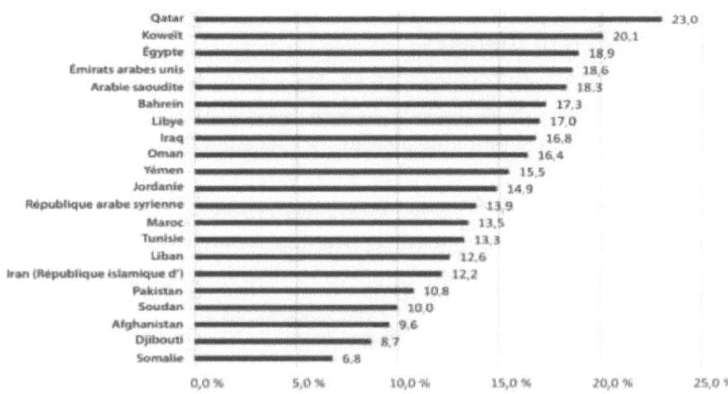

Figure 3: Age-standardised prevalence of diabetes by country in the Eastern Mediterranean region (2)

In sub-Saharan Africa, the current prevalence of diabetes is just 4.3%. However, the number of undiagnosed diabetics is 81.2%, and this figure is set to rise over the next 20 years. The situation is also alarming in the countries of the Middle East and the Gulf. Among the top ten countries with the highest prevalence of diabetes, six have the highest diabetes-related mortality rate in the world. For example, the prevalence of diabetes is around 24% in Saudi Arabia, 17% in Qatar, 14.1-16.1% in Oman and 13.4% in Jordan (27).

2.1.3.3. Prevalence of diabetes in Algeria

A study carried out in western Algeria in the Tlemcen region revealed that in a sample of 7,656 individuals, 36% of whom were men and 64% women, the overall prevalence of diabetes was 14.2%, with type 2 predominating in both urban and rural areas: the overall prevalence was 15.3% in urban areas and 12.9% in rural areas. The age distribution of diabetes in both sexes in the two settings shows that, overall, the age groups most affected are 30-39 and 40-49 (29).

Table 3: Breakdown of non-diabetics (type 1 and type 2) by gender (28)

Age group lans)	Urban environment									Rural areas						
	Men					Women			Men			Women				
	N/A	Type 1	Type 2	Total	ND*)	Type 1	Type 2	Total	ND*)	Type 1	Type 2	Total	N D	Type 1	Type 2	Total
20-29	160	3	31	194	550	15	29	594	112	9	16	137	255	5	16	276
30-39	225	11	43	279	234	35	49	318	203	13	62	278	277	5	37	319
40-49	214	35	44	293	491	30	40	561	246	12	46	304	595	19	47	661
50-59	195	15	59	269	405	18	30	453	148	8	17	173	316	12	31	359
60-69	145	7	69	221	285	9	31	325	152	5	19	176	378	8	43	429
>70	218	5	10	233	367	3	9	379	168	2	18	188	231	1	5	237
-Total	1 157	76	256	1 489	2 332	110	188	2 630	1 029	49	178	1 256	2 052	50	179	2 281

N.D*: Non-diabetics.

2.1.4. Complications of diabetes

Complications of diabetes are common and are responsible for considerable morbidity and mortality. Diabetes is one of the main causes of cardiovascular disease, blindness, kidney failure and lower limb amputations. It accounts for 10.7% of all-cause mortality worldwide (30).

Long-term complications of diabetes can be revelatory of the disease; in people living with undiagnosed T2DM, just as they can appear rapidly after the onset of T1DM. For this reason, early diagnosis is essential to prevent disability and death from diabetes (2).

2.1.4.1. Metabolic complications

Acute complications are the main cause of hospitalisation in diabetic patients, especially in emergency departments and intensive care units. The seriousness of these complications means that knowledge of their pathophysiology is essential for proper treatment (31) .

2.1.4.1.1. Hyperglycaemic complications

The two hyperglycaemic complications of diabetes are diabetic ketoacidosis (DKA) and hyperosmolar hyperglycaemia syndrome (formerly known as hyperosmolar coma), and their broadly similar pathophysiology means that the therapeutic approach to these two complications is almost identical: rehydration and insulin therapy (31, 32).

2.1.4.1.2. Lactic acidosis

Lactic acidosis is an organic metabolic acidosis due to an accumulation of lactic acid by an increase in its production or a decrease in its utilisation. Lactic acidosis occurs when blood lactate levels exceed 5 mmol/l (31). Lactic acidosis is the most serious complication of metformin treatment, with a mortality rate close to 50% (33); however, a recent meta-analysis found no difference in the incidence of this complication in diabetics treated or not treated with metformin (34).

2.1.4.1.3. Hypoglycaemia

Hypoglycaemia is an inseparable complication of diabetes treatment. Hypoglycaemia is the main factor limiting optimal control of diabetes. Damage to glucose counter-regulation mechanisms and the autonomic system increases the risk of severe hypoglycaemia 25-fold in insulin-treated T1DM and T2DM (35) . Its diagnosis is based on Whipple's triad, characterised by an abnormal drop in venous glycaemia, the presence of neuroglycopenic symptoms and their disappearance when sugar is taken. Hypoglycaemia in diabetic patients is defined as a capillary blood glucose level of less than 3.9 mmol/l (35). Preventing hypoglycaemia is crucial, and involves identifying risk factors and providing individualised education for each patient (35).

2.1.4.2. Chronic complications

Whatever its type, diabetes can lead to complications that affect several parts of the body and increase the overall risk of premature death. These include myocardial infarction, stroke, kidney failure, leg amputation, blindness and nerve damage. During pregnancy, poorly controlled diabetes increases the risk of intrauterine death (26).

The complications of diabetes can be classified as microvascular or macrovascular. Microvascular complications include damage to the nervous system (neuropathy), renal system (nephropathy) and eyes (retinopathy). Macrovascular complications include cardiovascular disease (36).

2.1.4.2.1. Macro angiopathy" cardiovascular complications

The atherosclerosis of the large and medium-sized arteries encountered in diabetes is known as macro-angiopathy. This atherosclerosis is not specific to diabetes, but it is characterised by its early onset, its multiple locations (coronary arteries, cerebral arteries, peripheral arteries) and its progression. The fact that it is often insidious and not very symptomatic means that it is often diagnosed late, which contributes to the severity of the prognosis (6).

Cardiovascular disease (CVD) accounts for up to 65% of all deaths in people with T1DM and T2DM (37). Ischaemic heart disease and stroke account for the largest proportion of morbidity associated with diabetes, and numerous prospective and retrospective epidemiological studies worldwide show that diabetes increases the risk of cardiovascular morbidity and mortality (2). Mortality rates due to heart disease are 2 to 4 times higher in diabetics than in non-diabetics (6).

2.1.4.2.2. Diabetes-related ocular complications

Diabetes-related eye diseases are particularly dreaded complications of diabetes, and essentially include diabetic retinopathy (DR), diabetic macular edema, cataracts and glaucoma, but also diplopia and inability to focus (2).

DR is defined, diagnosed and treated exclusively on the basis of the extent of retinal vasculopathy (38). DR is one of the main causes of blindness in the working population, with terrible personal and socio-economic consequences, despite being potentially preventable and treatable (1).

2.1.4.2.3. Nephropathy :

Chronic kidney disease (CKD) in people with diabetes can lead to ND or result from other associated diseases such as hypertension, neurogenic bladder, increased incidence of recurrent urinary tract infections or macro angiopathy (2). Worldwide, more than 80% of end-stage renal disease is caused by diabetes, hypertension or a combination of the two (2).

Diabetes, hypertension and CKD are intimately linked. In T2DM, hypertension often precedes CKD and contributes to the progression of kidney disease, whereas in T1DM, hypertension is more often a consequence of CKD. Diabetes and CKD are strongly associated with CVD, so controlling blood glucose and blood pressure can reduce the risk of CVD and CKD (2).

Table 4: Prevalence of diabetes complications (38)

	Neuropathy (various definitions)		Nephropathy (overt)		Retinopathy		Coronary heart disease	
Region	Min	Max	Min	Max	Min	Max	Min	Max

Africa	27.6	31.2	5.3	23.8	15.1	55.4	n.a.	na.
East Mediterranean and Middle East	21.9	56.0	6.7	6.7	14.4	64.1	15.0	19.8
Europe	16.8	33.7	7.6	15.0	11.3	44.7	3.3	25.2
North America	28.5	47.6	6.1	6.1	28.5	62.1	9.8	43.4
South and Central America	n.a.	n.a.	11.3	11.3	n.a.	n.a.	n.a.	n.a.
South-East Asia	12.7	15.0	3.8	3.8	11.0	30.2	2.0	33.7
Western Pacific	7.3	44.0	1.0	57.1	21.0	48.6	1.0	31.1
Overall	7.3	56.0	5.3	23.8	11.0	64.1	1.0	43.4

n.a. noi available.

Source. *Diabetes abas (59)*

2.1.4.2.4. Neuropathy :

Detectable sensory-motor polyneuritis occurs within ten years of the onset of diabetes in 40-50% of people with T1DM or T2DM (39).

Peripheral neuropathy is the most common form of diabetic neuropathy. It affects the distal nerves of the lower limbs, particularly those of the feet. This mainly alters sensory function symmetrically, leading to abnormal sensations and progressive numbness (38) .

Lower limb amputations in people with diabetes are ten to twenty times more common than in people without diabetes (2).

2.1.4.3. Other complications

2.1.4.3.1. Oral and dental complications

Diabetes has a negative impact on all the soft and hard tissues around the teeth. Compared with non-diabetics, several studies highlight the decisive role played by the severity of hyperglycaemia (28). Glycation inhibits the release of interleukin-10 (IL10) and tumour necrosis factor-alpha (TNF-α) from lymphocytes and macrophages. Unbalanced diabetics experience serious oral problems such as premature tooth eruption, gingivitis and periodontitis, as well as more caries, peri-implantitis, thrush, candidiasis and oral cancer, all of which can seriously compromise quality of life (2).

2.1.4.3.2. Erectile dysfunction :

Erectile dysfunction (ED) affects around 34-45% of men with diabetes. It has been shown to have a negative impact on the quality of life of men of all ages. In addition, studies indicate that 40% of diabetic men over the age of 60 have complete ED (39).

Ejaculation disorders are another common sexual dysfunction in diabetic men, occurring in up to 32% of cases. Hypogonadism is more common in diabetic men than in the general population (39).

2.1.4.3.3. Skin complications

A single recent prospective European study estimated the mean prevalence of skin complications during the course of DM (infectious or non-infectious and excluding the diabetic foot) at 54% of T1DM patients and 61% of T2DM patients. The prevalence of non-infectious dermatoses during the course of DM was studied in a recent prospective French study and was estimated at 56% of T1DM patients compared with 70% of T2DM patients (40).

2.1.5. Diabetes and covid 19

2.1.5.1. Introduction

The most common COVID-19-related comorbidities were hypertension, diabetes, CVD and diseases of the respiratory system (40). However, people with DM are exposed to greater severity and mortality than people without diabetes: 2.12 times mortality, 2.45 times severe COVID-19, 4.64 times acute respiratory distress syndrome (ARDS) and 3.33 times disease progression (41).

Table 5: Prevalence of comorbidities associated with COVID-19 (46)

	CMJ Hubei MC[1]	lancet Wuhan SC[1]	Lancet Wuhan DC	Lancet Wuhan SC	lancet Wuhan SC Severe Cases	NEJM S52 Hospitals	Pre-print 575 Hospitals	Lancet Wuhan DC	JAMA Wuhan SC	Allergy Wuhan SC
Follow-up time	12.30-1.24	"1.2	12.20'1.23	1.2'1.25	12.24'1.26	12.11'1.31	12.21'1.31	12.29-1.31	1.1'23	1.16'2.3
Number of cases	137	41	81	99	52	1099	1590	191	138	140
Severe	137(100%)	13(32%)	/	/	52 (100%)	173 (15.74%)	254 (16%)	119 (62.3%)	36(26%)	58 (41.4%)
Died	16(11.7%)	/	3(4%)	11 (11%)	32 (61.5%)	15 (1.4%)	/	54(28.3%)	6 (4.3%)	/
Chronic medical illness	27 (19.7%)	13 (32%)	21(26%)	50(51%)	21 (40%)	261(23.7%)	399 (25.1%)	91(48%)	64 (46.4%)	90(64.3%)
Cardiovascular & cerebrovascular diseases[1]	>13 (>9.5%)	>6 (>15%)	>12 (>15%)	40(40%)	>7 (>135%)	>165 (>15%)	>269 >16.9%)	>58(>30%)	>43 (>31.2%)	>42 >30%)
Diabetes	14 (10.02%)	8(20%)	10 (12%)	12 (12%)	9(17%)	81 (7.4%)	130 (8.2%)	36 (19%)	14 (10.1%)	17 (12.1%)
Digestive & endoain system disease}	/	/	/	>13 (13%)	/	/	/	!	/	>13 (9.3%)
Carcinoma	2(1.5%)	1(2%)	4(5%)	1(1")	2(4%)	10 (0.9%)	130(8.2%)	2(1%)	10(7.2%)	/
Chronic lung disease	2(1.5%)	1(2%)	9(11%)	1(1")	4(8%)	12 (1.1%)	24(1.5%)	6(3%)	4 (2.9%)	/
Chronic kidney disease	/	/	7(9%)	/	/	23 (2.1%)	28(1.8%)	2(1%)	4 (2.9%)	8(5.7%)
Chronic liver disease	/	1(2%)	3(4%)	/	/	8(0.7%)	21(1.3%)	/	4 (2.9%)	2 (1.4%)

2.1.5.2. Diabetes and covid19

Diabetes essentially appears to be a prognostic factor in the severe form of the disease. In a study of 201 COVID-19 patients, the prevalence of diabetes was 19% in patients hospitalised in an intensive care unit for severe pneumonia, compared with 5.1% in those requiring only hospitalisation in a non-intensive unit. In the same study, the prevalence of diabetes was 25% in patients who died (42).

Preliminary data from England from the National Health Service, available online but not yet published in a scientific journal, suggest that the risk is higher in people with T1DM compared with T2DM (43) .

Two recent UK studies report a positive correlation between increased risk of death and high HbA1C levels (43): diabetic patients with HbA1c >10% (86 mmol/mol) had a higher risk of COVID-19-related in-hospital death than those with HbA1c 6.5-7% (48-53 mmol/mol) (42). These data suggest that good control of diabetes prior to infection has a role to play in the prognosis and course of COVID-19. Indeed, a high HbA1c level is associated with inflammation, hypercoagulability and low SaO2 in patients with COVID-19, and the mortality rate (27.7%) is higher in diabetic patients (41).

2.2. Type 2 diabetes

The prevalence of T2DM is rising rapidly worldwide. Apart from the notion of an ageing population, this increase is the result of the interaction of several phenomena: genetic predisposition, epigenetic mechanisms, partly linked to an unbalanced, unhealthy diet in pregnant women, which has an impact on in utero programming; limited or even non-existent physical activity, over-consumption of energy-dense foods favouring the onset of overweight and obesity, not to mention possible exposure to various pollutants toxic to the ß-cell (44-46).

T2DM is a public health concern because of the worrying increase in its prevalence. It is now present in almost all populations, and epidemiological data suggest that failure to comply with the effective prevention and control programmes outlined by the WHO is likely to result in a very marked increase in its incidence (47, 48).

T2DM is particularly difficult to treat in patients under 25 years of age, for whom complex phenotypes may require several decades of intensive management to minimise the development and progression of microvascular and macrovascular complications (49).

The prevalence of T2DM increases sharply with age. Elderly people with type 2 diabetes are particularly fragile, as they combine the effects of ageing and the disease (49).

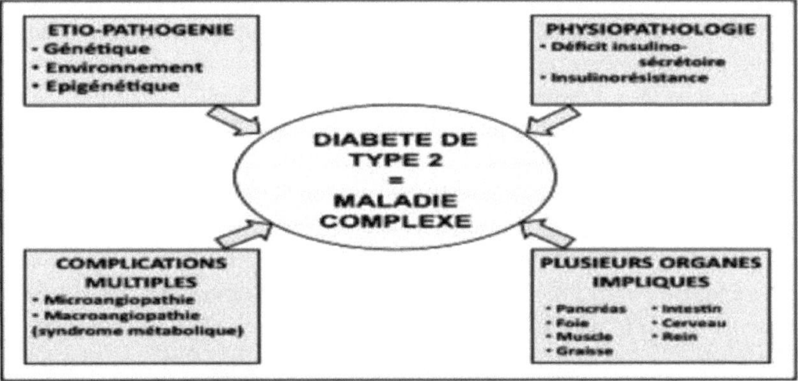

Figure 4: The complexity of type 2 diabetes in its different aetiopathogenic, pathophysiological and clinical components (6)

2.2.2. Pathophysiology of type 2 diabetes

T2DM is linked to alterations in insulin secretion favoured by older insulin resistance.

2.2.2.1. Alterations in insulin secretion

Alterations in insulin secretion are the common denominator of all forms of diabetes. They are grouped together under the term insulin dysfunction: abnormalities of pulsatility, abnormalities of kinetics, qualitative abnormalities, quantitative

abnormalities and progressive abnormalities. Insulin levels depend not only on insulin secretion, but also on insulin clearance, which is impaired in T2DM. Most of this clearance occurs in the liver (50).
Insulin levels should be compared with blood glucose levels. In a normal subject, insulin levels are multiplied by 2 or 3 when blood glucose is experimentally raised to 120 mg/dl, and by 10 for a blood glucose level of 225 mg/dl. The HOMA (homeostasis model assessment) index can help with this confrontation (51).

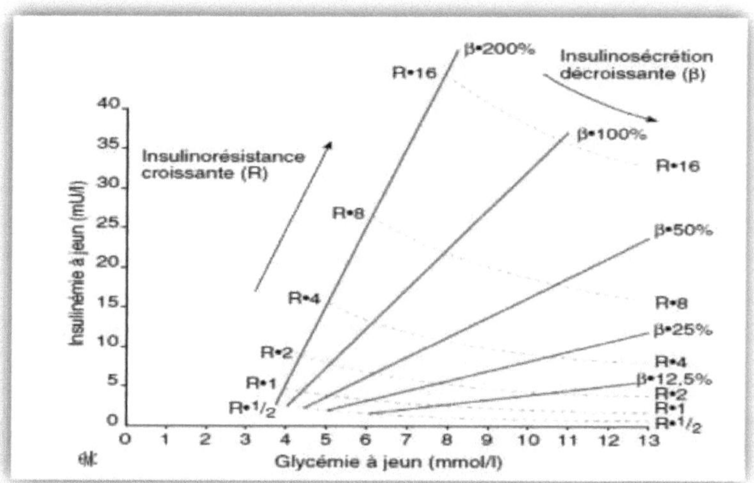

Figure 5: The HOMA model (57)

In T2DM, there is a reduction or disappearance of the rapid oscillatory secretion of insulin, which is one of the components of island dysfunction. On the other hand, there is abnormal hypersecretion of proinsulin and immature peptides, such as 32-33-cleaved proinsulin, which account for 40% of the peptides secreted by the cell, compared with 5% in non-diabetic controls. This may explain the state of hyperinsulinism in T2DM (52).
This functional defect would then be accompanied by a reduction in the total mass of beta cells, which would contribute to the development of the disease: in fact, a 65% reduction in the total mass of pancreatic beta cells is associated with T2DM (3).

2.2.2.2. Insulin resistance

Insulin resistance is defined as a reduction in the activity of insulin in the target tissues (muscle, liver and adipose tissue), more specifically a reduction in its action in inhibiting endogenous production and stimulating peripheral glucose utilisation (52, 53).
At the level of the adipocyte, the consequences of this insulin resistance are an increase in plasma concentrations of free fatty acids, which stimulate the neoglucogenesis and triglyceride synthesis. On the other hand, there is an increase in

the secretion of adipocytokines (TNF-α, interleukin 6, resistin) which inhibit the insulin signalling pathway. On the other hand, secretion of adiponectin (another adipocytokine) is reduced, as the latter stimulates muscle use of glucose via the AMPK (MP-activated protein kinase) pathway (52, 53). Another incriminating factor is the accumulation of free fatty acids in muscle, which modifies glucose metabolism, principally its intracellular penetration and catabolism, and disrupts insulin secretion (52-54).

On the other hand, prolonged exposure of the ß-cell to hyperglycaemia and high concentrations of triglycerides and free fatty acids leads to a progressive and irreversible reduction in the insulin secretion induced: hence the notion of glucotoxicity and lipotoxicity. But the real impediments to insulin action are located downstream of its receptor, inside the target cells. Negative control of the insulin signal may result from degradation of the hormone or dephosphorylation of its receptor, but above all it will result from phosphorylation of the serine/threonine residues on the receptor and insulin receptor substrate proteins. This phosphorylation can be activated by a number of pathological factors involved in insulin resistance, such as hyperinsulinism, TNFa or free AGs (53, 55).

These mechanisms may explain the insulin resistance induced by TNF-α, free fatty acids and glucocorticoids and therefore play an important role in the link between obesity and insulin resistance (the intracellular accumulation of ceramides and sphingolipids synthesised in excess from long-chain saturated fatty acids) (53, 56).

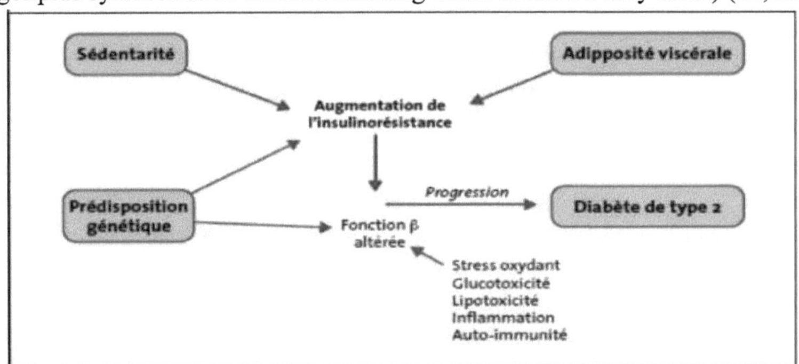

Figure 6: progressive and complementary pathophysiological mechanisms involved in type 2 diabetes (55)

Insulin resistance can also be explained by impaired glucose utilisation and glucose resistance. Impaired glucose utilisation in ß-cells can lead to a reduction in their insulin secretion (53, 57).

Physiologically, once present in the cell, glucose must be phosphorylated in the form of glucose-6-phosphate in order to be metabolised. Insulin resistance has a negative impact on the expression of hexokinases present in T2DM muscles (47).

However, oxidation and storage are not the only possible outcomes for glucose; the pentose pathway, 2-3% of glucose, can be used to synthesise hexosamines such as glucosamine, whose adverse effects on insulin action and secretion constitute an important mechanism of 'glucotoxicity' (53).

2.2.2.3. Inflammation of the islets of Langerhans

The involvement of islet inflammation in β-cell dysfunction in T2DM is now clear. Islet cells, including β-cells, play an important role in the initiation of islet inflammation, as they have the ability to sense stimuli and secrete chemokines as well as human islet amyloid polypeptid to activate macrophages (58).

Macrophages are the main source of pro-inflammatory cytokines in islets of Langerhans. Among these pro-inflammatory cytokines, IL-Iβ secreted by M1-type macrophages plays a crucial role in the initiation and amplification of inflammation in islets of Langerhans. In contrast, M2-type macrophages are essential for the development of islets of Langerhans and β-cell proliferation in humans (59, 60).

A better understanding of the role of macrophages in islet physiology may help to optimise strategies targeting IL-1. Given that inflammatory pathological changes have only been observed in a proportion of patients with T2DM, the identification of biomarkers correlated with islet inflammation will help to improve effective therapeutic prescription targeting islet inflammation by enabling appropriate patient selection, without systematically suppressing M1-type macrophages (58).

2.2.3. Risk factors for T2DM :

A better understanding of the natural history of T2DM opens up new prospects for preventing this complex disease (44).

The risk factors for T2D involve a combination of genetic and metabolic factors that contribute to its prevalence:

- Non-modifiable factors include ethnic origin, family history, gestational diabetes and advanced age.
- Modifiable factors include obesity, unhealthy diet and level of physical activity, all of which can contribute to the development of T2D.

Table 6: Modifiable and non-modifiable risk factors and their association with T2D(47)

Modifiable risk factors	Non-modifiable risk factors
Overweight* and obesity† (central and total)	Ethnicity
Sedentary lifestyle	Family history of Type 2 diabetes
Previously identified glucose intolerance (IGT and/or IFG)	Age
Metabolic syndrome:	Gender
Hypertension	History of gestational diabetes
Decreased HDL cholesterol	Polycystic ovary syndrome
Increased trigylcerides	
Dietary factors	
Intrauterine environment	
Inflammation	

*World Health Organization (WHO) criteria define overweight as a BMI ≥ 25 kg/m² [50].
†WHO criteria define obesity as a BMI ≥ 30 kg/m² [50]. For country/ethnic specific values for waist circumference as a measure of central obesity see table 4.
HDL, high-density lipoprotein; IFG, impaired fasting glucose; IGT, impaired glucose tolerance.

2.2.3.1. Non-modifiable factors

2.2.3.1.1. Genetics

T2D is linked to a strong genetic predisposition. It has not yet been possible to identify with certainty the genes linked to this susceptibility. Understanding the differences between ethnographic groups exposed to similar environments implies a significant genetic contribution (47) .

2.2.3.1.2. Age

The prevalence of type 2 diabetes increases markedly with age. The age of onset of the disease has shifted towards young adults and even adolescents in recent decades, particularly in countries where there is a significant imbalance between energy intake and expenditure (47).

2.2.3.1.3. Previous gestational diabetes

In the case of gestational diabetes, glucose tolerance generally returns to normal after delivery. However, these women have a significantly higher risk of developing T2DM later in life (47).

2.2.3.2. Modifiable factors

2.2.3.2.1. Obesity

The respective prevalences of obesity and type 2 diabetes continue to rise throughout the world, reaching unprecedented levels. The reasons for this rapid increase remain complex, and for the moment there is no clear-cut answer. The existence of a positive energy balance resulting from overeating, combined with a sedentary lifestyle, are obviously the two key factors in the development of insulin resistance, along with a genetic predisposition, as shown by family studies and studies of monozygotic twins, with highly variable degrees of involvement (61).

In addition to the severity of excess weight, the type of body fat distribution plays an important role, in particular the accumulation of fat in the abdominal area (62).

Insulin resistance is the key element linking obesity to diabetes: adipose tissue is now considered to be a metabolically active endocrine organ capable of producing substances that modify insulin sensitivity and are implicated in the metabolic syndrome: free fatty acids, pro- or anti-inflammatory cytokines (61, 62).

2.2.3.2.2. HTA

Hypertension is associated with T2DM in 80% of cases; it is more frequent, particularly in elderly diabetics. This combination of hypertension and diabetes is responsible for an increased cardiovascular risk, with the onset of cardiovascular morbidity and accelerated deterioration in renal function.

The combination of hypertension and diabetes is a public health problem because of its chronicity, the difficulty of treating it and the seriousness of its complications (63).

These two pathologies each constitute a cardiovascular risk factor with a cumulative effect (64).

In T2DM, insulin resistance plays an important role in the pathogenesis of increased blood pressure. Very often, hypertension is associated with diabetes and sometimes precedes its diagnosis. Hypertension and diabetes interact to accelerate arterial ageing. In the context of T2DM, the aetiology of the increase in

arterial pressure is mainly due to excess weight, hyperinsulinism, insulin resistance with activation of the sympathetic system, stimulation of the renin angiotensin system, water retention and endothelial lesions in the microcirculation (65).

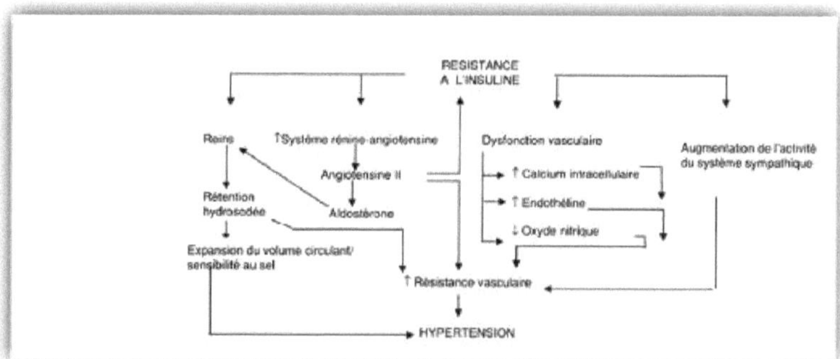

Figure 7: Pathogenesis of hypertension in the context of insulin resistance (65)

2.2.3.2.3. DYSLIPIDEMIA

Lipid abnormalities are frequent and specific to type 2 diabetes patients. They are defined by high levels of triglycerides (large VLDL particles rich in triglycerides), a change in the composition of LDL (dense and small), low levels of HDL-C (enrichment of HDL with triglycerides) and qualitative abnormalities in atherogenic lipoproteins (glycation of apolipoproteins).

These abnormalities are likely to favour the onset of cardiovascular accidents, due to their atherogenic nature (66).

Dyslipidaemia affects almost 50% of T2DM patients and increases the risk of cardiovascular disease in patients who are already at high cardiovascular risk. Disruption of lipid metabolism appears to be an early event in the development of T2DM, and may precede the disease by several years (67).

2.2.3.2.4. Smoking

Smoking is a well-known major cardiovascular risk factor. Despite the identification of several health-damaging pharmacological agents in the composition of tobacco, no clear explanation has been reported for its link with all the pathogenic effects. It is also possible that certain components of tobacco are toxic to the B cells of the islets of Langerhans in the pancreas (68-70).

Cessation of tobacco consumption leads fairly quickly to a correction of various biological anomalies often encountered in the presence of insulin resistance: it improves glycaemic control in type 2 diabetic patients in the short term and also reduces the cardiovascular risk in diabetic patients (70).

Smoking leads to sympathetic hyperactivation, which is responsible for an increase in pulse and blood pressure on the one hand, and a rise in circulating catecholamine concentrations on the other. Catecholamines are powerful insulin antagonists and can induce a state of insulin resistance. Attvall *et al.* have also demonstrated a significant increase in another hormone involved in glycaemic counter-regulation, growth hormone (GH), during cigarette smoking (70, 71).

2.2.3.2.5. Physical activity

The role of a sedentary lifestyle in the onset of T2D has been suggested for many years. Epidemiological data strongly support the role of physical activity in the prevention of obesity and T2D. Sedentary behaviour, on the other hand, has received less attention (72).

Regular physical activity increases the sensitivity of peripheral tissues to insulin and improves the mechanisms controlling glymoregulation. In addition to its built-in hypoglycaemic effect, physical activity promotes weight loss and/or weight stabilisation, even in the elderly (17).

Da Qing's study is based on an increase of one unit per day of leisure-time physical exercise. The results on the incidence of glucose intolerance-DT2 conversions were clear, falling from 15.7% of subjects per year in the control group to 8.3 in the group subjected to physical exercise alone. In patients of normal weight, the incidence of glucose intolerance-DT2 conversions was 13.3% in the control group and 5.1% in the group subjected to the physical exercise programme (17).

Table 7: Definition of a "physical exercise unit" according to the study by DA QING (20)

Intensité	Durée (min)	Nature
Doux	30	Marche lente, courses dans les magasins, nettoyage de la maison
Modéré	20	Marche rapide, descente d'escaliers, danse (lente), bicyclette
Intense	10	Course lente, montée des marches d'escaliers, danse (disco), volley-ball, tennis de table
Epuisant	5	Saut à la corde, basket-ball, natation.

2.2.4. Type 2 diabetes and metabolic syndrome

The metabolic syndrome (MetS) is characterised by an aggregate of metabolic disorders whose coexistence in the same individual may correspond to a common pathophysiological mechanism, on the one hand, and expose the subject to an increased risk of subsequent onset of T2DM and cardiovascular disease, on the other (73, 74). DM is increasingly considered to be a major public health problem (75).

2.2.4.1. Definition of DM

The WHO has proposed a definition of this syndrome, thereby legitimising its role in public health. According to the definition adopted by the National Cholesterol Education programme Adult Treatment Panel , an individual is a carrier of this syndrome when he or she presents at least three of the following five risk factors:

1. Abdominal obesity defined as a waist circumference >102 cm in men and >88 cm in women;
2. A rise in fasting triglycerides >150 mg/dl;
3. A reduction in HDL cholesterol <40 mg/dl in men and <50 mg/dl in women;
4. An increase in blood pressure >130/>85 mm Hg;
5. A rise in fasting blood glucose >110 mg/dl.

According to the IDF, a person with DM must have at least two other factors among those already included in the definition of the National Cholesterol Education program Adult Treatment Panel II (73, 75). This new definition of DM therefore places the emphasis on abdominal adiposity (75).

2.2.4.2. Etiopathogenesis

The causes of SM are multifactorial, with three main origins: genetic predisposition, *in utero* determinism and environmental influence (73).

2.2.4.2.1. Genetic predisposition

It is generally accepted that around 25% of individuals in the general population have reduced insulin sensitivity, regardless of the presence of obesity. The causes of this anomaly are still poorly understood, and the origin is probably polygenic. This genetic predisposition will be expressed more or less early depending on exposure to environmental risk factors (73).

2.2.4.2.2. In utero determinism

Epidemiological studies have shown that people with low birth weight have a higher risk of developing DM, hypertension and T2DM. Low birth weight for gestational age reflects delayed growth *in utero*, generally associated with placental underdevelopment. This situation favours metabolic adaptation *in utero* that persists into childhood, adolescence and adulthood.

Placental underdevelopment predisposes to insulin resistance and to diabetes mellitus, which is assimilated to T2DM in men (75, 76).

2.2.4.2.3. Environmental factors

Environmental factors play a major role. This is the case for a sedentary lifestyle and an unbalanced, unhealthy diet responsible for excess weight and then obesity. Finally, stress and smoking also aggravate insulin resistance (77). For people with DM, the risk of developing T2D is particularly high in subjects with abdominal obesity (73).

CHAPTER 3

2.3. Diabetic nephropathy (DN)

CKD comprises a group of conditions in which renal excretory function is chronically compromised, mainly as a result of damage to kidney structures.

Most, but not all, forms of CKD are irreversible and progressive. Kidney damage includes :

- Loss of nephrons due to deletion of glomerular or tubular cells.
- Fibrosis affecting both glomeruli and tubules.
- Impaired renal vascularisation.

CKD is a frequent complication of diabetes, hypertension, nephritis, inflammatory and infiltrative diseases, renal and systemic infections (streptococcal infections, bacterial endocarditis, human immunodeficiency virus -HIV-, hepatitis B and C), polycystic kidney disease, autoimmune diseases (systemic lupus erythematosus), renal hypoxia, trauma, nephrolithiasis and lower tract obstruction, chemical toxicity or others (78).

Whether it is glomerular, tubular or renal-vascular involvement, the chronic course eventually converges towards common histological and functional alterations of the kidney affecting most renal structures, leading to progressive and generalised fibrosis and glomerulosclerosis (78). Once established, CKD can be diagnosed consistently, whatever its cause (79).

2.3.1. Definition of ND

Diabetes is associated with 40% of new cases of end-stage renal disease and is the leading cause (7) .

MRD includes typical ND and other forms of kidney damage(16).

ND is known as Kimmelstiel-Wilson syndrome, nodular diabetic glomerulosclerosis or inter-capillary glomerulonephritis. It is a clinical syndrome characterised by albuminuria (>300 mg/day or >200 mg/min) confirmed on at least two occasions 3-6 months apart, a permanent and irreversible reduction in GFR and hypertension (80).

The syndrome was first described by the British physician Clifford Wilson (1906-1997) and the American physician Paul Kimmelstiel (1900-1970) in 1936 (81).

Renal disease in diabetics is one of the chronic complications of microangiopathy. It is a glomerular disease. It is the leading cause of dialysis initiation in developed countries, and its prevalence is increasing (from 25 to 50%) in parallel with the rise in the prevalence of T2DM. Diabetic dialysis patients have a two-fold increase in the risk of cardiovascular death compared with non-diabetic dialysis patients, and a 100-fold increase compared with the general population. Patients with ND have a very high cardiovascular risk comparable to the cardiovascular risk of patients with coronary heart disease (12, 82), which is in direct competition with the risk of kidney damage (8, 80).

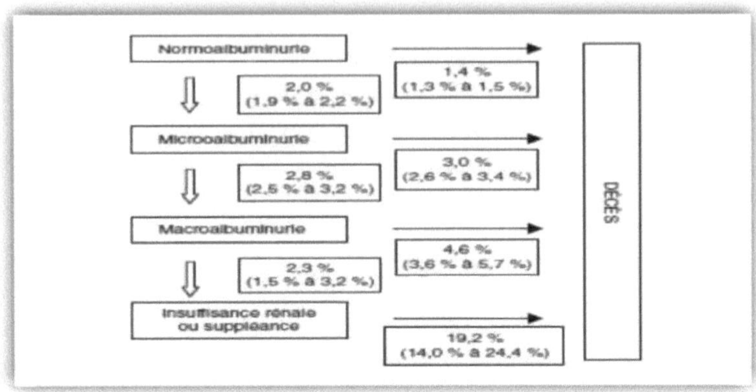

Figure 8: Annual transition rates from one stage of kidney disease to the next, and competitive mortality rates for each stage of kidney disease in the UKP study (8)

2.3.2. Epidemiology

In patients with CKD, the prevalence of ND was 30.3%, followed by chronic interstitial nephritis (23%) and chronic glomerulonephritis (17.7%) (83).

Approximately 20-30% of patients develop microalbuminuria after 15 years of disease, and less than half develop full-blown nephropathy (84).

The European Diabetes Prospective Complications Study Group (EURODIAB) and the Danish 18-year study have shown that the overall incidence of microalbuminuria in patients with T1DM and T2DM is 12.6% and 33%, respectively (12).

Proteinuria develops in around 15% to 40% of patients with T1DM, generally after 15 to 20 years of diabetes (81). In patients with T2DM, the prevalence varies between 5% and 20% on average (80).

If left untreated, the delay between the onset of incipient nephropathy (microalbuminuria) and the onset of CKD is 10 to 15 years. This means that CKD occurs on average 25 years after the diagnosis of diabetes. ND is more common in African-Americans, Asians, Amerindians and Hispanics than in Caucasians. Scientists have not been able to explain these higher rates and the interaction of the various risk factors (83).

Compared with Caucasians, patients from South-East Asia have a higher prevalence of proteinuria and a lower prevalence of microalbuminuria. This would suggest that progression to CKD is more rapid in subjects from South-East Asia (85). Fortunately, this trend is declining, most likely due to better prevention and earlier diagnosis and treatment of DM (81).

According to the ENTRED 2007 study, the glomerular filtration deficit estimated by the simplified MDRD formula was greater than 90 ml/min/1.73 m^2 for 23% of T2DM, between 60 and 90 ml/min/1.73 m^2 for 43% of diabetics, and less than 60 ml/min/1.73 m^2 for 19% of diabetics. This calculation was impossible for 15% of patients in the

population studied (86, 87).
In our region of North Africa, it accounts for 11-18% of the causes of end-stage renal failure (88). In Algeria, its frequency is estimated at 20% in diabetics of all types (89).

2.3.3. Pathophysiology

The pathophysiology of ND can be roughly divided into two parts
There is a complex interaction between metabolic and haemodynamic disturbances (90, 91).

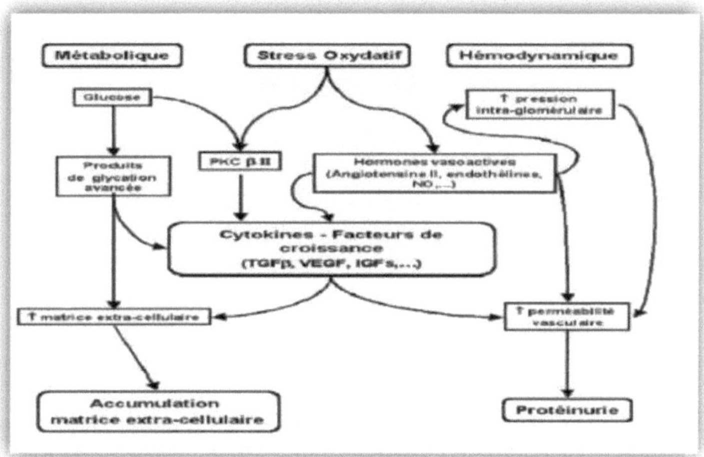

Figure 9: Pathophysiology of diabetic nephropathy (103)

2.3.3.1. The role of hyperglycaemia and oxidative stress

In ND, the metabolic alteration induced by hyperglycaemia is at the heart of the development and progression of ND and therefore the appearance of characteristic renal lesions (85, 92), which include thickening of the glomerular basement membrane, mesangial expansion and the appearance of characteristic Kimmelstiel-Wilson nodules.

The concept of glucotoxicity covers several mechanisms:

J Non-enzymatic glycation of proteins leading to advanced glycation products (AGEs) which also induce TGF-β, a profibrogenic cytokine.

J The feeding of the polyol pathway by excess glucose, with the formation of sorbitol and then fructose, which exert an osmotic stress effect.

J Incomplete glycolysis, which provides substrates for the hexosamine pathway, the end products of which stimulate, among other things, the production of TGF-ß via protein kinase C (PKC); the increase in flux via the hexosamine pathway leads to an increase in the expression of up Stream stimulating factors (USSF), which trans-activate the TGF-ß promoter.

J The auto-oxidation of glucose to keto-aldehydes with the production of free radicals which, together, damage proteins (90, 93).

Hyperglycaemia leads to the formation of AGEs, which bind to collagen in the glomerular basement membrane and to mesangial and endothelial cells and podocytes. The consequences of AGE generation are the production of various cytokines, inflammatory factors and cell growth factors, such as VEGF (vascular endothelial growth factor) and TGF-β (transforming growth factor beta), resulting in expansion of the mesangial matrix, glomerulosclerosis and increased urinary albumin excretion (94).

At vascular level, hyperfiltration with endothelial dysfunction is observed in ND, notably in relation to the production of nitric oxide (NO) under the action of endothelial nitric oxide synthase (ENOS). One hypothesis is that the accumulation of AGEs disrupts the ENOS enzyme and alters the production and availability of NO. This leads to endothelial dysfunction at the glomerular level and therefore a defect in autoregulation, which contributes to the development of ND (94).

On the other hand, the generation of free radicals by oxidative stress pathways is increased by hyperglycaemia and will provoke excess production of cytokines and growth factors, maintaining the inflammatory phenomenon of ND and leading to expansion of the mesangial matrix and a pro-fibrotic state (94-96).

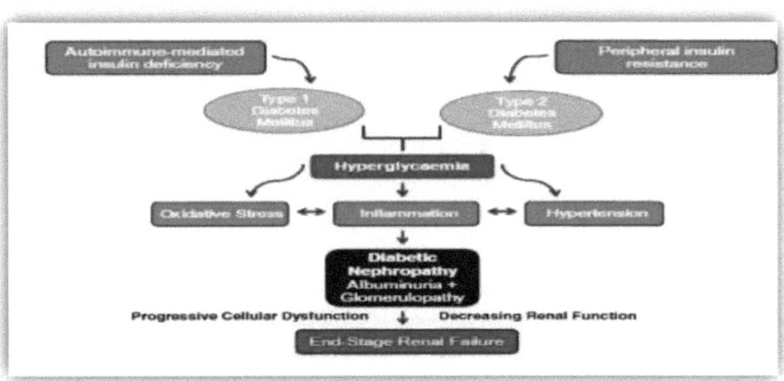

Figure 10: Role of hyperglycaemia in the development and progression of diabetic nephropathy (112)

Abnormal signalling in ND is caused by the transforming growth factor (TGF-1). TGF-βI expression is elevated in a variety of kidney cells.

Dysfunctional TGF-βI signalling modulates glucose flux in renal cells by upregulating the glucose transporter, GLUT-1. SMAD (similar protein of mothers against decapentaplegic) proteins are effectors of intracellular TGF-βI signalling due to their ability to translocate to the nucleus and regulate transcription (97, 98).

The relevance of the TGF/SMAD pathway in the development of diabetic glomerulosclerosis and tubulointerstitial fibrosis has been demonstrated using animal models.

Beyond this well-known pathway, recent research has demonstrated the existence of a complicated crosstalk between TGF1ß- and other well-known non-SMAD pathways (99).

2.3.3.2. Intra-renal haemodynamics

Other critical mediators of ND include haemodynamic elements, such as activation of vasoactive hormonal pathways, most commonly the renin-angiotensin-aldosterone system (RAAS) (85, 99).

At various stages in the development of ND, changes in intra-renal haemodynamics may be observed, in particular an increase in intra-glomerular pressure.

The initial phase of hyperglycaemia leads to preferential vasodilatation of the afferent arteriole, which is clinically manifested by glomerular hyperfiltration.

Glomerular hyperfiltration is a well-characterised consequence of early-onset diabetes; globally, it is observed in 10-40% of patients with T1DM and up to 40% of patients with T2DM (90). The mechanisms involved in glomerular hyperfiltration in diabetes are incompletely understood, however, one plausible mechanism is an increase in proximal tubular reabsorption of glucose by the sodium-glucose cotransporter 2, which decreases the distal supply of solutes, particularly sodium chloride, to the macula densa. The consequence of the reduction in tubulo-glomerular feedback is dilation of the compensatory afferent arteriole, leading to an increase in glomerular perfusion. At the same time, high local production of angiotensin II in the efferent arteriole produces vasoconstriction. The overall effect is elevated intraglomerular pressure and glomerular hyperfiltration (100) .

This hyperfiltration can lead to an abnormal leakage of proteins into the urine, known as microalbuminuria (30 to 300 mg of albumin in the urine/day). Initially, the amount of protein is minimal, but over time and depending on the extent of kidney damage, proteinuria can increase considerably, reaching up to 300 mg of albumin in the urine per day, known as "macro albuminuria"(94).

2.3.4. History of the disease :

ND is one of a group of microangiopathies characterised by involvement of small vessels less than 30 µm in diameter (101).

The natural history of development, in 3 phases and 5 stages, was described by Mogensen towards the end of the 1980s (7).

In the early phase, there is hypertrophy of the glomeruli and proximal tubules, leading to glomerular hyperfiltration (102).

J **The second phase** is characterised by hypertrophy of the mesangium linked to an increase in the extracellular matrix and the number of mesangial cells, and a thickening of the glomerular basement membrane. This second phase corresponds to a state of glomerulosclerosis.

J **The next phase** is characterised by a progressive reduction in capillary density, a change in the size of the pores of the glomerular basement membrane and a reduction in the filtration surface area (7).

In the early stages of ND, increased kidney size and changes in Doppler indicators may be the first morphological signs of kidney damage, while proteinuria and GFR are the best indicators of the degree of damage (81) .

Stage 1: Corresponds to a phase of renal hypertrophy and hyperfiltration. It is characterised by glomerular hyperfiltration present from the onset of diabetes and an increase in the size of both kidneys.

Stage 2: In the majority of cases, this is a latent or silent phase. It begins a few years after the onset of diabetes and may persist for several decades. It is characterised by the appearance of minimal histological lesions in the kidney, which have no clinical significance. Many patients remain at this stage for the rest of their lives.

Stage 3: is characterised by the appearance of signs of incipient nephropathy after at least 5 years of diabetes, but more often after 10 to 20 years. It affects 30 to 40% of T1DM. It is defined by the presence of microalbuminuria corresponding to an increase in EUA of more than 30 mg/24 h but less than 300 mg/24 h (or > 20 mg/L but < 200 mg/L).

Stage 4: Clinical patent nephropathy, with macroscopic proteinuria in excess of 300 mg/24 h (detected by urine dipstick) and CKD with reduced GFR and hypertension.

Stage 5: Corresponds to pre-terminal or terminal IR, an irreversible state leading to replacement therapy with iterative dialysis and/or transplantation. Proteinuria decreases and renal function collapses. If left untreated, this stage occurs 10 to 15 years after the onset of stage 3 (103-105).

Table 8: Classification of renal damage according to MOGENSEN (118)

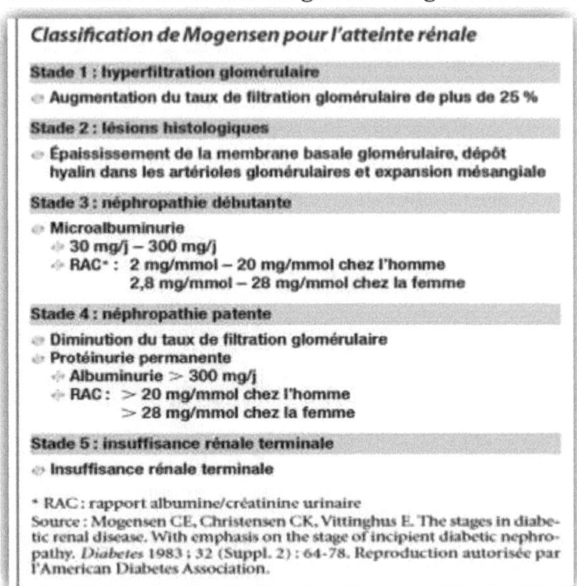

Classification de Mogensen pour l'atteinte rénale

Stade 1 : hyperfiltration glomérulaire
- Augmentation du taux de filtration glomérulaire de plus de 25 %

Stade 2 : lésions histologiques
- Épaississement de la membrane basale glomérulaire, dépôt hyalin dans les artérioles glomérulaires et expansion mésangiale

Stade 3 : néphropathie débutante
- Microalbuminurie
  - 30 mg/j – 300 mg/j
  - RAC* : 2 mg/mmol – 20 mg/mmol chez l'homme
    2,8 mg/mmol – 28 mg/mmol chez la femme

Stade 4 : néphropathie patente
- Diminution du taux de filtration glomérulaire
- Protéinurie permanente
  - Albuminurie > 300 mg/j
  - RAC : > 20 mg/mmol chez l'homme
    > 28 mg/mmol chez la femme

Stade 5 : insuffisance rénale terminale
- Insuffisance rénale terminale

* RAC : rapport albumine/créatinine urinaire
Source : Mogensen CE, Christensen CK, Vittinghus E. The stages in diabetic renal disease. With emphasis on the stage of incipient diabetic nephropathy. *Diabetes* 1983 ; 32 (Suppl. 2) : 64-78. Reproduction autorisée par l'American Diabetes Association.

Source: Mogensen CE. Christensen CK, Vittinghus E. The stages in diabetic renal disease. With emphasis on the stage of incipient diabetic nephropathy. *Diabetes* 1983; 32 (Suppl. 2): 64-78. Reproduced with the permission of the American Diabetes Association.

Renal involvement in T2DM is much more heterogeneous:

S Only 1/3 of patients develop lesions characteristic of diabetic glomerulosclerosis in isolation.

S 1/3 of patients have predominant vascular lesions of the fibrous endarteritis type (nephro-angiosclerosis);

S 1/3 do not have diabetic disease, but have other types of nephropathy or nephropathy in addition to diabetic lesions, justifying a renal biopsy.

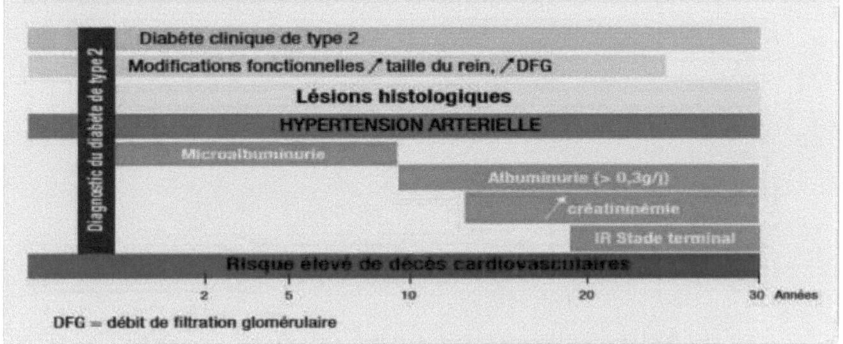

Figure 11: Natural history of nephropathy in T2DM (8)

2.3.5 Risk factors

MRD risk factors can be classified conceptually as follows:

J Susceptibility factors (age, gender, race or ethnicity, and family history),

J Initiation factors (hyperglycaemia) and progression factors (hypertension, diet and obesity),

The two main risk factors for developing DRD have been identified as hyperglycaemia and hypertension. There is undoubtedly an individual susceptibility to the development of ESRD, given that it affects only around 40% of diabetic subjects, even in the presence of glycaemic or blood pressure imbalance. There is also a family history of diabetes with nephropathy (16, 95).

2.3.5.1. Hyperglycaemia

Metabolic memory" suggests that early and intensive glycaemic control can prevent irreversible damage such as epigenetic alterations associated with hyperglycaemia (106).

In patients with T1DM, an intensive glycaemic control intervention aimed at achieving HbA1C < 7% as a therapeutic goal reduced the 9-year risks of microalbuminuria and macroalbuminuria by 34% and 56% respectively, compared with standard care. The intensive therapy group had approximately 50% low GFR 60 ml/min /1.73 m^2 , and the mean rate of decline in GFR was significantly reduced from 1.56 ml/min /1.73 m^2 per year with standard treatment to 1.27 ml/min / 1.73 m^2 per year with intensive treatment (16).

Table 9: Risk factors for ND (16)

Initiateurs

- Hyperglycémie chronique avec mémoire métabolique
- Rôle de la prédisposition génétique:
  - agrégation familiale de ND
  - gènes candidats (par exemple: polymorphisme gène ACE I/D, NO synthase)
  - analyse complète du génome
- Rôle de l'épigénétique:
  - méthylation de l'ADN
  - modification des histones de la chromatine
  - micro ARN et ARN longs non codants
- Influence ethnique: prédisposition accrue chez les Noirs, Asiatiques et/ou Hispaniques

Promoteurs de progression

- Hyperglycémie, durée du diabète (> 10 ans)
- Obésité et syndrome métabolique
- Hypertension artérielle
- Tabagisme
- Hyperlipidémie (cholestérol et triglycérides)
- Albuminurie

Similarly, in newly diagnosed T2DM patients, after ten years of intensive glycaemic control intervention aiming for an HbA1C < 6% resulted in a 24% reduction in the development of microvascular complications, including MRD, compared with the results observed after conventional treatment (100).

Inadequate glycaemic control is a key risk factor for the development and progression of ND. Elevated HbA1c levels have been associated with an increased risk of kidney disease in people with both T1DM and T2DM.

Patients who already had moderate albuminuria but low HbA1c levels had a reduced risk of developing severe albuminuria or ESRD in the Diabetes Control and Complications Trial/Epidemiology of Diabetes Interventions and Complications (DCCT/EDIC) trial (16). Randomised controlled trials in patients with T1DM and T2DM have shown similar results. Intensive glycaemic management reduced the likelihood of progressing from moderate to severe albuminuria or ESRD in the DCCT study. However, it is not certain that the various anti-diabetic drugs are all equally effective (12).

1.1.5.2. Urinary excretion of albumin

It is a marker and a major factor in the progression of kidney damage. Increased albumin excretion in the urine is a major risk factor for the progression of ND in both T1DM and T2DM.

The first symptom of ND is a moderate increase in EUA in the majority of individuals. More specifically, 30 to 300 mg/g of creatinine in a morning urine sample (also known as microalbuminuria) (107).

Patients who develop a significant increase in albuminuria, defined as >300 mg albumin/g creatinine in a morning urine sample (also known as macro albuminuria) have a particularly high risk of deterioration in renal function. However, a significant proportion of patients with moderate albuminuria (around 40%) return to normal albuminuria (108).

Furthermore, despite the presence of mild albuminuria or even normo albuminuria, up to 50% of patients with T1DM or T2DM experience a decrease in GFR deficit (109). Therefore, a high AUE is not a necessary condition for the development of ND. This has implications for the diagnosis of the disease, namely that GFR should be assessed in addition to EUA (12).

1.1.5.3. HTA

Hypertension is another important independent risk factor for kidney disease. In the DCCT/EDIC study, low blood pressure was associated with a low probability of progressing from moderate albuminuria to severe albuminuria or CKD (110) .

In addition, blood pressure reduction was associated with a regression from moderate to normo albuminuria in patients with T2DM. Inhibitors of the renin-angiotensin system appear to slow the progression of ND more than other antihypertensive drugs, while lowering blood pressure in a similar manner (111).

T1DM patients with proteinuria are hypertensive: elevated blood pressure is a consequence of nephropathy. However, any prior hypertension is a risk factor for the onset and acceleration of the early stages of nephropathy (8). Each 10 mm Hg increase in systolic blood pressure has been linked to a 15% increase in the risk of developing micro- and macro-albuminuria, as well as impaired renal function defined as a GFR of 60 ml/min/1.73 m^2 or a doubling of blood creatinine (112).

In general, a systolic pressure of 140 mm Hg has been linked to a higher risk of ESRD and death in people with T2DM (113).

All interventional studies have clearly established that optimal blood pressure control is capable of reducing the rate of progression of lesions and RI (12).

1.1.5.4. Dyslipidaemia

There is no clear evidence that dyslipidemia is predictive of the development of ND. Low levels of low-density lipoprotein cholesterol (LDL-C) and triglycerides (TG) were observed in the DCCT/EDIC study. However, albuminuria was found to decrease in diabetics taking the statin. Interventional studies using statins are underway to try to prove that correcting these abnormalities would be able to slow the progression of renal disease (114).

High levels of total cholesterol (TC) have also been associated with an increased likelihood of developing moderate to significantly enlarged UA in patients with T2DM. Furthermore, in T2DM, low TC and TG levels are associated with a regression from moderate to normo albuminuria (12).

1.1.5.5. Tobacco

Smoking has been found to be an independent risk factor for the development of albuminuria in non-diabetic adolescents. A recent study of people with kidney disease, hypertension and controlled diabetes receiving optimal insulin therapy found that 53% of smokers developed a severe form of their kidney disease, compared with only 11% of non-smokers (68).

The effect of smoking could amplify that of poor glycaemic control, by reducing the ability of the vascular wall to adapt to the metabolic and haemodynamic stresses associated with chronic hyperglycaemia (68).
In addition to controlling blood pressure and glucose levels, it is therefore essential for diabetic patients to limit their tobacco consumption (8).

1.1.5.6. Obesity

Obesity is also associated with an increased risk of ND (115). In the DCCT study, abdominal obesity, as assessed by waist circumference, was associated with a higher incidence of albuminuria, but did not predict a decline in GFR. In contrast, weight loss reduced EUA and prevented a decline in GFR (111).

1.1.5.7. Age and sex

In both T1DM and T2DM, advanced age increases the risk of nephropathy. This link appears to be independent of the duration of diabetes. In the DCCT/EDIC study, female gender was associated with a low risk of progression from mild to severe albuminuria and even ESRD (111).

1.1.5.8. Retinopathy

In individuals with T1DM, the development of retinopathy almost often precedes the development of nephropathy. In the DCCT/EDIC study, the absence of retinopathy was associated with a low risk of moderate and severe albuminuria and even ESRD. In T2DM, more than half of individuals with kidney disease have no retinopathy unless the kidney disease is caused by diabetes (12, 116, 117).
In the same patient, retinopathy always precedes the clinically evident signs of kidney disease. Although a small proportion of individuals with advanced retinopathy have glomerular histological changes and microalbuminuria, the majority of patients with advanced retinopathy have no obvious signs on renal biopsy; in patients with T2DM, the association between ND and retinopathy is weak (118).
Biopsy was performed on 36 patients with T2DM and kidney disease in the study by Schwartz *et al.* In 17 cases, biopsy revealed obvious glomerulosclerosis with Kimmelstiel-Wilson nodules, while in the other 15 cases, biopsy revealed alterations compatible with ND (mesangial sclerosis), but no typical nodules. There was no difference in the duration of disease progression or glycaemic control between patients with and without nodules. A substantial association was found between severe retinopathy and the presence of Kimmelstiel-Wilson nodules. The explanation for this phenomenon is still unknown (81).
The Wisconsin epidemiological study (Klein 1984), which included 1,370 diabetics diagnosed before the age of 30, found a prevalence of diabetic retinopathy ranging from 28% to 77% depending on whether diabetes had been present for 5 or 15 years. The severity of this retinal disease is related to the value of glycated haemoglobin, the increase in systolic blood pressure and the presence of proteinuria (119).

1.1.5.9. Genetics

A large number of new genes have been discovered, thanks in particular to the resurgence of genome-wide association studies (GWAS). This research has proved to be an effective tool for determining the genetic architecture of ND. However, the GENIE consortium has recently demonstrated the limitations of this genome-wide approach (120).

Although this is the largest genome-wide association study focused on ND to date, it has highlighted the great complexity of ND inheritance and identified new genes. The genes identified are probably responsible for only a limited proportion of the phenotypic alterations observed in diabetic patients with kidney disease. Furthermore, it is possible that the pathogenic pathways differ between T1DM and T2DM ND (99).

An investigation was carried out on a set of 66 diabetic germline pairs which were found to be incompatible with the nephropathy disease. A linkage disequilibrium was found between a region of the long arm of chromosome 3, which includes the angiotensin type 1 receptor (AT1R) gene, and ND. However, an in-depth study of the AT1R gene revealed no significant polymorphisms associated with nephropathy.

The two main pathophysiological axes which have justified the study of candidate genes in ND concern the metabolic and haemodynamic hypotheses (121).

1.1.5.9.1. Genes involved in the metabolic pathway

The link between nephropathy and glycaemic imbalance prompted researchers to discover possible genes involved in increasing or decreasing sensitivity to hyperglycaemia. The role of sorbitol and aldose reductase in diabetic problems was discovered through research into metabolic pathways. Genetic polymorphisms affecting this enzyme have been linked to diabetic retinopathy and have recently been discovered in ND (121).

Another area of research into the metabolic hypotheses involved in diabetic pathophysiology concerns redox and the production of AGEs (122). Genetic polymorphisms have been described in the gene encoding the AGEs receptor. The different functional aspect of the AGEs receptor seems to be able to modulate the tissue consequences of the redox and glycation phenomena involved in the genesis of ND (123, 124).

1.1.5.9.2. Genes involved in the haemodynamic pathway

The haemodynamic pathophysiological hypotheses concern the hypertension genes, because of the more frequent family history of subjects with nephropathy than those without, and also because of the deleterious effect of arterial hypertension on the development or worsening of diabetic nephropathy (121).

The genes of the renin angiotensin aldosterone system have been particularly well studied: The angiotensin-converting enzyme (ACE) gene is therefore a logical candidate gene, especially as ACE levels are familial segregated and an insertion/deletion (I/D) polymorphism in intron 16 of the ACE gene, 287 base pairs in length, is associated with variable ACE levels in T1DM (125, 126). Other studies have suggested that polymorphisms in the angiotensin II receptor, aldose reductase and protein kinase C may also play a role in the progression of ND (12).

Another approach was to assess the degree of renal damage in subjects who had already expressed a major risk of microangiopathy complications (retinopathy). In this cross-sectional study strategy, the effect of the ACE I/D genotype revealed the existence of an interaction between this polymorphism and the M235T polymorphism of the angiotensinogen gene. The renin gene polymorphism and genes for extracellular matrix components are candidate genes for the development of glomerulosclerosis (124).

1.1.5.10. Other factors

Oxidative stress and subclinical inflammation both appear to contribute to the pathogenesis of ND.

Patients with T1DM or T2DM who have elevated levels of pro-inflammatory cytokines and chemokines (interleukin-6, interleukin-18, monocyte protein-1 or chemoattractant-1), HS-CRP or adhesion molecules have a higher risk of developing nephropathy and progressing to more severe kidney disease (12). Patients with T1DM or T2DM have an elevated number of tumour necrosis factor receptors, which are associated with an increased prevalence of renal dysfunction (12).

CHAPTER 4

2.4. Other diabetic kidney diseases

The aetiological assessment of diabetic nephropathy is critical, as it is necessary to distinguish "classic" diabetic nephropathy from chronic nephropathy of vascular, glomerular or congenital origin, as well as from glomerulonephritis, which is increasing rapidly (7).

Although there is no pathological microalbuminuria, a significant number of diabetics have impaired renal function (GFR <60). The specific nature of the renal lesions in these individuals, which are very probably non-glomerular, has not been studied in depth, but they appear to be less progressive.

However, pathological microalbuminuria does not always imply the presence of glomerular disease in T2DM patients. Their renal biopsies may be normal (1/3), or show a predominance of tubulointerstitial and vascular lesions (1/3), rather than typical glomerular disease (1/3) (127).

Apart from ND (65% of cases), around 7% of T1DM patients on dialysis in France in 2006 had vascular nephropathy, 5% had glomerulonephritis, and 22% had an unknown aetiology (6). Only around 10% of patients had a repeat biopsy, so these results should be interpreted with caution. Apart from ND (53% of cases), approximately 20% of T2DM dialysis patients in France in 2006 had vascular nephropathy, 4% had glomerulonephritis and 21% had unknown aetiology (87).

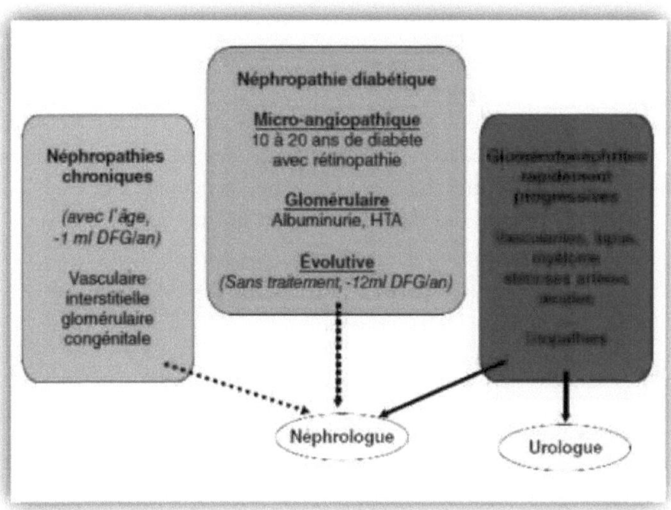

Figure 12: Renal damage in patients with T2DM: diagnostic hypotheses

(139)

2.4.1. Ischaemic nephropathy :

Caused by atherosclerotic changes in the small and large renal arteries, ischaemic nephropathy can lead to chronic kidney disease in diabetics. Ischaemic nephropathy is characterised by low GFR and, in most cases, low albuminuria (sometimes non-existent). According to a series of kidney biopsies carried out on T2DM patients, non-diabetic glomerulopathy (ischaemic nephropathy) is as common as chronic kidney disease in type 2 diabetes. Clinical studies appear to show that between 25% and 50% of diabetics with significant renal dysfunction do not have albuminuria (128).

Table 10: Clinical and biological factors that distinguish classic diabetic nephropathy from other kidney disorders (134)

Facteurs susceptibles d'orienter le diagnostic vers la néphropathie diabétique classique plutôt que vers d'autres troubles rénaux	
Néphropathie diabétique	**Autre trouble rénal**
Albuminurie persistante	Protéinurie extrême (> 6 g/jour)
Sédiment urinaire inactif	Hématurie (microscopique ou macroscopique) persistante ou sédiment urinaire actif
Évolution lente de la maladie	Baisse rapide du DFGe
Faible DFGe associé à une protéinurie patente	Faible DFGe avec protéinurie faible/absente
Présence d'autres complications du diabète	Absence d'autres complications du diabète ou complications relativement moins graves
Durée connue du diabète > 5 ans	Durée connue du diabète < 5 ans
	Antécédents familiaux de néphropathie non diabétique (p. ex., polykystose rénale)
	Signes ou symptômes d'une maladie systémique

2.4.2. Atherosclerotic stenosis of the main renal veins and branches

This is a common and sometimes overlooked feature of diabetic and non-diabetic patients with severe diffuse atherosclerosis. In around a third of cases, there is renal artery stenosis, which is associated with hypertension and/or impaired renal function. The recommended score for detecting renal artery stenosis is based on the presence of diffuse vascular disease, hypertension and an elevated blood creatinine level (129).

However, because several organs are frequently involved, diagnosis can be difficult. Renal infarction is a rare condition associated with stenosis of the main arteries. When a diabetic patient presents with a clinical picture that at first glance appears identical to that of acute pyelonephritis, this should be taken into account (130).

Table 11: Types of diabetes-related kidney damage (16)

Mécanismes de l'atteinte rénale dans le diabète
1. Néphropathie diabétique classique (glomérulosclérose diabétique) (figure 1) • Rôle métabolique : hyperglycémie • Rôle hémodynamique : – stimulation système RAA – hyperfiltration glomérulaire • Rôle inflammatoire Passage par les stades classiques : hyperfiltration, reins augmentés en taille, microalbuminurie (A2), macroalbuminurie (A3) avant la baisse du DFG
2. Athérosclérose de l'aorte et des artères rénales avec sténose éventuelle, néphroangiosclérose • Rôle des facteurs de risque classiques d'athérosclérose • Elévation des indices de résistances vasculaires intrarénales Baisse du DFG sans albuminurie ou avant l'apparition de celle-ci
3. Maladies tubulo-interstitielles • Conséquences d'infections urinaires • Toxicité médicamenteuse • Hyperuricémie Baisse du DFG sans albuminurie mais avec marqueurs urinaires d'atteinte tubulaire (alpha 1 microglobuline urinaire accrue)

In fact, many diabetic patients present a fall in GFR without albuminuria or retinopathy, especially, but not exclusively, in the context of T2DM.

2.4.3. Diabetic nephropathy with normo-albuminuria

A fall in GFR without proteinuria is observed in one-third to one-half of T2DM patients at some stage in the course of the disease. The common feature of these patients is a slower progression to CKD, which is associated with increased cardiovascular risk. This type of nephropathy is observed in elderly people who have had diabetes for several years, have a history of cardiovascular disease and are being treated with a renin-angiotensin system inhibitor (7).

Finally, in T2DM, kidney damage may develop at a "pre-diabetes" stage, although there is already evidence of kidney disease linked to insulin resistance (7). In the UK Prospective Diabetes Study (*UKPDS*), 51% of people who developed a creatinine clearance of 60ml/min/1.73m^2 tested positive for albuminuria (10). Some, but not all, observational studies show that a decline in GFR is slower in T2DM patients with low or normal albuminuria (7).

The absence of albuminuria in diabetics with reduced GFR raises the possibility of non-diabetic CKD. The NKF (national kidney foundation) KDOQI (national kidney disease outcomes quality initiative) working group on diabetes and CKD concluded that the presence of retinopathy in patients with CAR 300 mg/g creatinine was strongly suggestive of CKD, and its absence in those with CAR < 30 to 300 mg/g creatinine suggested non-diabetic CKD. These results were confirmed in a recent meta-analysis (131).

The NKF KDOQI diabetes guidelines and the *CKD* guidelines are particularly relevant for diabetics with normal levels of albuminuria and a GFR of 60 mL/min/1.73 m^2 (131). Measurement of albuminuria is not standardised and is imprecise; assays have recently been developed using isotope dilution mass spectrometry and have shown variations of around 40% compared with conventional assays (for albumin concentrations of 13 mg/L to 1084 mg/L) (131, 132).

Recommendations from the ADA, the NKF, and the National Kidney Disease Education Program (NKDEP) support measurement of albuminuria more than once and indicate that two of the three samples should be raised over a period of 3 to 6 months for confirmation of a diagnosis of albuminuria (132, 133). The take-home message from this study is the importance of following the trajectories of GFR decline and albuminuria in diabetics, an approach already advocated for diabetics before they reach stage 3 CKD (133).

CHAPTER 5

2.5. Markers of diabetic nephropathy

2.5.1. Former ND markers

ND affects almost a third of people with diabetes and is the main cause of ESRD in most countries. According to the recommendations of the *ADA* and the French Kidney Foundation, the fundamental markers for the detection and monitoring of CKD in diabetic patients are defined by the EUA level and the estimated GFR, which is poorly assessed by serum creatinine alone but estimated by the Cockcroft-Gault (CG) formulae or the Modification of Diet in Renal Disease (MDRD) (10, 134).

2.5.1.1. Determination of glomerular filtration rate

GFR is considered to be the best indicator of renal function, even though the physiology of the kidney is not limited to the filtration process. Normal' GFR is around 120 ml/min/1.73 m^2 . The progressive "physiological" loss of nephron mass is associated with an average decrease in GFR of around 0.5 - 1 ml/min/1.73 m^2 per year from adulthood onwards (135).

Creatinine, the product of muscle creatine metabolism, is the most widely used marker for estimating GFR. It is freely filtered at the glomerular level.

In addition to its exogenous "red meat" intake, creatinine is mainly produced by muscles and depends on muscle mass, which is higher in men and black individuals and decreases with age in adults (135) .

In a less restrictive way, certain drugs such as fibrates can have an impact on muscle creatinine production and on the accuracy of GFR estimates in diabetic patients (136).

Serum creatinine clearance, on the other hand, depends not only on the GFR but also on tubular secretion: in healthy people, creatinine clearance exceeds the GFR by 10%. This difference can reach +60% in nephropathies with severe proteinuria, such as nephrotic syndrome, when the level of serum creatinine exceeds the GFR.

apparently normal, masks obvious changes in GFR (137).

On the other hand, techniques for measuring creatinine have undergone major changes in recent years. The colorimetric method (Jaffé) is the most widely used, but lacks specificity (cross-reaction with other circulating chromogens). The enzymatic method is much more specific and has been recommended by the HAS (French National Authority for Health) since 2011, but its widespread use is limited by its high cost. Finally, since 2007, this assay has been standardised, using standards obtained by spectrometric method (IDMS), which guarantees reproducibility between automated systems (138).

These numerous influences make it necessary to estimate GFR, but they also raise questions about the validity of the formulae used in such a patient population (11) .

In response to this public health problem, the American NKF-KDOQI (National kidney foundation Kidney disease outcome quality initiative) and international KDIGO (Kidney disease improving global outcome) expert committees have issued recommendations for the systematic estimation of GFR in adults using the MDRD

(Modification of diet in renal disease) equation or the Cockcroft-Gault (C-G) equation (135).

> The Cockcroft-Gault (C-G) equation

The C-G equation is the most common and most widely used, particularly for adjusting drug dosage (135).the formula was developed with the aim of estimating creatinine clearance without the need for tedious and imprecise urine collection (139). This equation, published in 1976, was developed from a group of 249 Canadian subjects, mostly men, and uses creatinine clearance measured in the urine as the reference method. The equation takes into account age (year), weight (kg), sex (k men = 1.23; k women = 1.03), and serum creatinine (mmol/l). The main limitation of this equation is the importance of weight: the values may be distorted in extremely thin or extremely obese people (135). Theoretically, therefore, it tends to overestimate the true GFR because it takes into account tubular secretion of creatinine (139).

Table 12: Formulas used to calculate GFR (146)

Débit de filtration glomérulaire mesuré (Cl-créat) = (créatinine urinaire x débit urinaire)/ créatinine plasmatique
Formule de Cockcroft et Gault (CG) Homme = [(140-âge) x poids (kg) x 1,23]/créatinine (µmol/L) Femme = [(140-âge) x poids (kg) x 1,02]/créatinine (µmol/L)
Formule simplifiée MDRD ***(modification of diet in renal disease)*** $=175*(\text{créatinine } (\mu mol/L)/7\ 823)^{-1,154} \times \text{âge}^{-0,203}$ x 0,742 (si femme) x 1,21 (si race noire)
Formule de Hoeak *et al.* (eDFG) =-4,32+ (80,35/cystatine (mg/L))

> MDRD formula

The method used to derive the MDRD formulae was completely different. The aim this time was to predict GFR measured by a reference method. The group of American patients was mainly Caucasian (88%), with a mean age of 50.6 years; the majority had stage 3 to 4 renal failure (mean measured GFR of 39.8 ml/min/1.73 m^2), 6% of whom had diabetes. They had a body mass index of 28 kg/m2, were 60% male and 12% black (140).

Multiple regression incorporating a large number of variables has made it possible to derive several formulae of increasing complexity. The formula initially recommended is known as MDRD (139, 141). The reference GFR was measured by the clearance of 125 I-iothalamate. In 2000, the team of Levey et al. developed a GFR prediction equation based on serum creatinine and demographic data from the MDRD study (135).

The latest simplified version of the MDRD formula, known as the abbreviated version, uses only 4 parameters: sex, age, creatinine level and race. The GFR estimated by the MDRD equation is immediately indexed for body surface area (135) . More recently, a final modification has been made, allowing this formula to be used with a creatinine level standardised on the reference isotope dilution mass spectrometry (IDMS) creatinine assay method. As the majority of creatinine assay kits are connected to the IDMS method, this corrected version of the MDRD formula is currently the most widely used (139, 142). The so-called simplified or abbreviated MDRD formula is available in two versions: the original adapted to non-standardised creatinine levels, and the other modified to adapt to creatinine levels standardised on the IDMS (143).

> **Formula CKD-EPI (Chronic Kidney Disease Epidemiology)**

More recent, it is derived from the same parameters as the MDRD and established using the same reference method, with creatinine levels measured using the enzymatic method. Its main specificity is that it is modelled differently according to the value of creatinine, with the aim of improving the predictive performance of the MDRD formula above 60 ml/ min/1.73 m^2 (140).

It was derived from a much larger sample (5504 patients) with an average age of 47 years, an average body mass index of 28 kg/m^2 , 32% of whom were black, and an average GFR of 68 ml/min/1.73 m^2 . Like the MDRD formula, the complexity of the CKD-EPI formula requires a handheld computer or online calculator. The formula is standardised on body surface area (139, 140).

> **Formula performance and outlook**

Numerous studies have shown that the Cockcroft formula performs much less well than the MDRD and CKD-EPI (140) . Some studies have found that one or other formula is superior in certain populations (diabetics, obese, elderly subjects), although this superiority has often not been confirmed. Overall, the MDRD formula appears to perform slightly better than the Cockcroft formula in patients with CKD (140).

The only limitations of the latter 2 formulas are patients with a low BMI and, in the case of MDRD, an overestimation of GFR at low creatinine levels. CKD- EPI is most useful for high GFR values > 90 mL/min/1.73 m^2 , or even > 60 mL/min/1.73 m^2 , for which its specific modelling gives it greater accuracy (140).

The HAS and international guidelines stipulate that the Cockcroft formula should no longer be used to estimate GFR and recommend the use of the CKD- EPI formula, which has demonstrated the best performance over the entire GFR spectrum, as first-line treatment (144).

2.5.1.2. Estimation of urinary excretion of albumin

2.5.1.2.1. Definition

The term microalbuminuria (or pauci albuminuria) refers to urinary excretion of albumin in very small quantities, intermediate between physiological values of around 30 mg/24 h and frank proteinuria, in excess of 300 mg/24 h.

Albumin is a serum protein with a relative mass of 67 kDa. Its glomerular passage is very low compared to its serum level. Tubular reabsorption is rapidly saturable. Any increase in EUA therefore reflects glomerular dysfunction (tubular abnormalities can be detected by measuring ß2-M (145).

Microalbuminuria is not only a risk factor for nephropathy and kidney damage, but is also linked to a high risk of cardiovascular events and death, particularly in T2DM

(146).

In the general population, microalbuminuria is found in 5-10% of subjects. Here too, microalbuminuria is a predictive factor for early mortality, in association with cardiovascular risk factors similar to those for T2DM. More generally, microalbuminuria can have several meanings:

S Variations have been observed during physical exercise;

S There is an increase in congestive heart failure, urinary tract infections and, more generally, febrile episodes;

S In systemic lupus erythematosus, it may be a criterion for monitoring.

S Albuminuria concentration values can also be modified by orthostatism

S in elderly subjects without diabetes is predictive of coronary mortality and stroke (147, 148).

2.5.1.2.2. Microalbuminuria tests

There are several ways of collecting urine for albumin measurement:

J 24-hour urine; however, this type of collection is often difficult to carry out correctly. The result is expressed in mg/24 h.

J Urine sample: In the case of this procedure, the albumin assay must be combined with a creatinine assay to reduce the inaccuracy of the collection. The result is expressed in mg/g of urinary creatinine or mg/mol of urinary creatinine. Standardisation of both albuminuria and urinary creatinine assays is necessary to obtain comparable ACR values between the different methods and between the different laboratories.

J Minute urine sample and then the expression of the result is in µg/min.

For the last 2 types of urine sampling, it is preferable to have fresh urine collected in the middle of the stream (149).

However, there is currently no consensus on how urine should be collected: neither the type of sample, nor the time of day when it should be taken, although it is known that the time of day can affect the results, both for urine samples and for spot urine sampling (145).

Samples can be stored at 2-8°C for 7 days. However, there are many different recommendations for the long-term storage and stability of albumin in urine samples (150, 151). Recent data suggest that urine samples are stable at -80°C for long periods. Storage at higher temperatures, particularly -20°C, appears to induce variable changes in albumin (149, 151, 152).

Tableau 13 Definitions of microalbuminuria and reference values (28)

Collection	24-hour urine (mg/24 h)	Timed collection (mg/min)	Sample Albumin/creatinine ratio (mg/g)	Sample Albumin/creatinine ratio (mg/mmol)
Normoalbuminuria	<30	<20	<30	<2
Microalbuminuria	30-300	20-200	30-300	2-20
Macroalbuminuria (protein urea)	>300	>200	>300	>20

Microalbumin cannot be detected by simple test strips. Immunoassay is the technique of choice for measuring albumin in urine: immunoturbidimetry or

immunonephelometry. The results of the external assessment of *Probioqual* show that nephelometric assays give higher results than turbidimetry (153).
Assays using high-performance liquid chromatography (HPLC) coupled with mass detection seem to be reserved for the development of reference materials and reference techniques (154).
HPLC made it possible to detect ND on average 3.9 years earlier (155) than the results obtained by immunoassay. Other studies show that 15-30% of subjects considered normal with urinary albumin immunoassay are classified as having microalbuminuria by HPLC (24, 149).
Unlike other urinary biomarkers, urinary albumin has the advantage of being an automated assay, widely used in laboratories (145).

Tableau 14 Discordance between microalbuminuria detected by immunoassay and HPLC (28)

	HPLC>20mg/l and immunoassay < 20 mg/l	HPIC > 30 mg/g and immunoassay < 30mg/g
Witnesses	21/32 (65,6%)	20/29 (69%)
Diabetes	34/60 (56,7%)	32/60(53,3%)

2.5.1.2.3. Phantom albumin :

The quantity and molecular forms of albumin present in urine may differ from those present in plasma due to tubular filtration and reabsorption of modified forms of albumin, modification of albumin by proteolysis during passage through the urinary tract, chemical modification by oxidants, free radicals and other ligands present in urine, and modification during storage of the sample (149) .
In rodents, it has been described that albumin is metabolised during renal filtration, resulting in the excretion of a mixture of intact protein and fragments. The same phenomenon has been described in humans and attributed to a transformation of albumin by lysosomal enzymes located at the tubular level (156).
What's more, this degradation is thought to be exaggerated in diabetic subjects.
The urine therefore contains :
J An intact albumin with its disulphide bridges and reactive immunity;
J A modified albumin which has lost its epitopes and is therefore non-immune reactivates;
J Albumin fragments corresponding to chains cleaved by enzymatic action.
It is the evidence of the second form in many subjects that has led some authors to speak of "phantom" albumin (24).

2.5.1.2.4. Microalbuminuria: a biomarker of cardiovascular disease

There is a quasi-linear relationship between increased urinary protein excretion and myocardial infarction and stroke in patients with T2DM. These observations are also valid for non-diabetic patients (157).
Screening for albumin, or protein in the urine, (even at lower levels below 150 mg/d) can have significant predictive value in identifying patients who are more likely to

suffer a cardiovascular event (158).
The urine albumin/creatinine ratio (CAR) was found to have a gradual linear relationship with cardiovascular morbidity and mortality. Due to the large number of participants in the study, the researchers were able to observe a linear relationship between CAR and cardiovascular mortality well below the standard threshold for microalbuminuria (30 mg/g creatinine), indicating that screening should be carried out early so that preventive treatment can be planned to reduce cardiovascular risk (158).

2.5.2. New biomarkers

2.5.2.1. Cystatin C

In 1961, three different authors independently described a new protein using immunoelectrophoresis. Clausen and Mac Pherson observed this protein in the cerebrospinal fluid (CSF) of healthy patients but did not find it in the blood. Butler found this protein in the urine of 79% of 31 patients with tubular disease. He hypothesised that the protein originated in plasma, but that it simply could not be measured due to the lack of sensitivity of the technique. In electrophoresis, this alkaline, low-molecular-weight protein appears after the gamma globulin band, hence the first names given to it, such as "post-γ protein" or "γ trace" (159).
In 1979, Lofberg and Grubb of Lund University (Malmo, Sweden) described the measurement of this γ-trace protein by radial immunodiffusion with a detection threshold of 300 μg/L. They confirmed its presence in blood, saliva and CSF, but in different quantities; the concentration in CSF is 5 times higher than in plasma, which explains its initial discovery in CSF (159).
In three dialysis patients, the same authors found much higher serum concentrations than in healthy subjects, prompting them to suggest that it undergoes glomerular filtration and is catabolised at tubular level. It was only after its amino acid sequence and molecular weight (13260 Da) were described in 1982 that Brezin noticed the similarity between this protein and a cysteine proteinase inhibitor belonging to the cystatin family. This was later confirmed by Barret and Grubb, who renamed the γ-trace protein "cys C" (159, 160).

2.5.2.1.1. Definition and characteristics

Cys C is a basic (pH 9.3), non-glycosylated polypeptide composed of 122 amino acids with a molecular weight of 13 kDa. It belongs to the family of cysteine proteinase inhibitors. Cys C is constantly synthesised and secreted by all the nucleated cells in the body (161). The gene coding for the protein is one of the housekeeping genes, whose expression is continuous (161). The production of cys-C is little influenced by sex, muscle mass, age or diet (159, 162).
Its level in the blood does not vary throughout the day. Its low molecular weight and positive charge allow it to be freely filtered at the glomerular membrane. It is then reabsorbed and completely catabolised by the cells of the proximal tubule, without secretion or reabsorption of the intact form (163).
The plasma concentration of Cys-C appears to depend mainly on GFR, but it is nevertheless possible that variations in production influence its concentration. In fact,

one study recently suggested that thyroid function may modify Cys-C production. It has been shown that thyroid hormone levels are inversely correlated with serum creatinine levels, but directly correlated with cys-C levels (164). Consequently, when cys C levels are considered, glomerular filtration rate is most likely overestimated in hypothyroidism and underestimated in hyperthyroidism (164).
Urinary cys-C concentration is very low, except in cases of proximal tubular damage (159).

2.5.2.1.2. Dosage methods and reference values

It was not until 1994 that rapid, fully automated methods were developed, all based on liquid agglutination of latex particles coated with polyclonal antibodies directed against cys C (163).
Methods for measuring cys C have gradually improved (more accurate, rapid and automated). Currently, this molecule is measured using the PETIA (particle-enhanced turbidimetric immunoassay) or PENIA (particle-enhanced nephelometric immunoassay) technique (165).
The essential technical difference between the two methods lies in the fact that PETIA can be performed on a multiparametric biochemistry machine (wavelength of around 340 to 650 nm depending on the application) whereas PENIA, which requires an infrared wavelength, can only be performed on a machine dedicated to immunonephelometry (159).
Two types of calibration equipment are used:
J The DakoCytomation and Gentian AS applications use human serum devoid of Cys C and enriched with recombinant Cys C.
J The Siemens application uses purified urinary Cys C. Immunonephelometric applications are only available on immunonephelometers in the BN® range from Siemens and the IMMAGE range from Beckman-Coulter (160).
At the Cantonal University Hospital in Geneva, using the nephelometry technique (PENIA), they mentioned the existence of interference with the PETIA technique (underestimation of cys C in the event of bilirubin >100 mg/l or triglycerides > 15g/l). On the other hand, no interference has been described with the PENIA method. However, calibration has not yet been standardised and this method is not available on most automatic analysers (159-161).
The reference values for cys C are 0.70-1.21 mg/l (before age 50) and 0.84-1.55 mg/l (after age 50), but these have not yet been standardised (159).
Most authors also describe a trend towards higher reference values for cys C after the age of 50-60 years (given the decrease in GFR with age (-12 ml/min/10 years after 50 years). Paediatric values are currently being validated (165).

2.5.2.1.3. Cys C stability

The stability of cys-C in serum has been studied in 3 main studies. They suggested that cys-C was stable at room temperature for 7 days, at -20°C for 1 to 2 months and at -80°C for at least 6 months and even several years. It was also shown that freeze/thaw cycles had no effect on cys-C (159, 163).

2.5.2.1.4. Cys C GFR marker

Several studies have validated the use of cys C as a renal marker in adults. Grubb *et al* (30) found that cys-C and creatinine correlated similarly (r 0.77 and 0.75, respectively) with GFR calculated by 51Cr-EDTA (chromium-51 ethylenediaminetetraacetic acid) Clearance in 135 individuals (aged 7-77 years) with a variety of kidney diseases, including primary kidney disease as well as secondary glomerulonephritis, rheumatoid disease and ND (166).

In two studies involving a total of 469 people, Newman *et al* (19, 32) concluded that, as well as being a better marker of GFR estimation than creatinine, cys C was a more sensitive marker of moderate changes in GFR than Cr. When the 206 renal patients were analysed separately, the correlation between Cys C and GFR (determined by 51Cr EDTA clearance) was r= 0.80, which was significantly better than the correlation with Cr (r= 0.50). These studies show that Cys C has been shown to be as effective as creatinine as a renal marker in the adult population. The majority of these studies even show a superiority of cystatin C. This last feature has made the study of cys C more attractive in particular populations (166).

In recent years, cys-C has emerged as an alternative filtration marker to creatinine. Its production is constant over time, independently of age, sex and muscle mass. It is freely filtered in the glomerulus and then completely degraded in the proximal tubule, so is not excreted. Its plasma concentration is inversely proportional to GFR (167) (168).

The performance of formulae derived from cys-C alone is no better than that derived from creatinine in the general population. On the other hand, this marker is probably of interest in subpopulations where muscle production of creatinine is very different from the population of the same age and sex, which accounts for the very poor performance of formulae derived from plasma creatinine (169).

Lastly, formulae incorporating both creatinine and cys C have been proposed which perform significantly better than those derived from creatinine alone in the general population (168).

For this reason, it is interesting to examine these different studies according to the sub-population studied:

> Paediatric population

Serum creatinine levels in children vary with age, height and weight due to changes in muscle mass. Filler (170) was the first researcher to study 216 children with a normal GFR (determined by EDTA-Cr51) and showed that plasma cys C levels did not vary with age (at least not for more than one year). This was later confirmed by other teams who demonstrated the independence of cys C from weight, height and sex in children (unlike creatinine). The reference values for cys-C in children over the age of four are more or less the same as those described for adults (166).

Premature babies, newborns and children under the age of four have higher cys-C values. Data on the relationship between plasma cys-C concentration and GFR in children are fragmentary and contradictory (159, 165).

> Kidney transplant patients :

Early detection of a decline in GFR, suggesting the possibility of acute rejection, is an essential element in the follow-up of a kidney transplant patient. This is particularly important in the first few weeks after transplantation (171).

The first study in kidney transplant patients showed that the determination of plasma cys-C concentration was superior to serum creatinine, with inulin clearance used as the reference. However, the number of patients studied was small (n = 12) and children were also included (159, 160, 165).

> Acute and chronic renal failure and diabetes:

Since the GFR determined from creatinine is overestimated due to the secretion of creatinine by the tubular cells, plasma creatinine is not sufficiently sensitive to detect incipient CKD of various origins (hypertension, diabetes, etc.).This is because cys-C levels begin to rise at a glomerular filtration rate of less than 88ml/min/1.73m^2 , whereas creatinine levels only become pathological when the GFR falls below 75ml/min/1.73m^2 (171).

Cys C is also undeniably useful in cases of acute renal failure (ARF). Cys C measurement enables AKI to be diagnosed 48 hours before plasma creatinine. Cys C therefore appears to be an interesting marker in the diabetic population for the detection of early nephropathy (162).

> Elderly subjects :

In practice, the estimation of renal function in elderly subjects is based on the determination of creatinine and the predictive equations derived from this. However, age-related sarcopenia leads to a drop in creatinine production. The Cockcroft and Gault formula systematically underestimates GFR in the elderly. However, the MDRD, which is more reliable, can only take into account an average age-related fall in muscle mass and creatinine (160).

Inflammation, malnutrition and muscular deconditioning can further accentuate abnormalities in muscle metabolism and affect the value of predictive equations based on creatinine. Cys-C may therefore appear to be an alternative marker; in the elderly, Cys-C appears to be less sensitive to metabolic and extrarenal factors than creatinine. It appears to be a promising marker for early detection of renal dysfunction in the elderly (160).

> Hepatocellular failure:

Cirrhotic patients represent a population for which measurements of plasma creatinine and creatinine clearance do not correlate well with GFR because of the interference of bilirubin in creatinine measurement, the extent of amyotrophy, which is very common in this condition, and possibly a decrease in the liver's capacity to convert creatine into creatinine. According to Woitas and Demirtas , the correlation coefficient with GFR assessed by a reference isotope approach for plasma cys-C is significantly higher than for creatinine (166). In these patients, cys-C has been shown to be equivalent to creatinine for assessing renal function, and even superior (159).

> Cystic fibrosis and neoplasia :

There are two reasons to monitor renal function in cancer patients undergoing chemotherapy:

S Direct damage to the renal tubules secondary to chemotherapy.

S Significant accumulation of these drugs and their metabolites when GFR is reduced.

When the GFR is 60 ml/min/1.73 m^2 , for example, the dose of cisplatin should be halved. Therefore, it should be advantageous to detect changes in renal function as early as possible (166).

Cys C is a major inhibitor of cathepsins, enzymes capable of proteolysis of the extracellular matrix and therefore of facilitating the degradation of basal membranes by tumour cells, and hence the metastatic process. The anti-tumour effect of Cys-C could also be based on a "*cytokine-like*" role independent of its function as a protease inhibitor(159). Plasma Cys-C concentration does not appear to be significantly influenced by a neoplastic process (165).

> Cys C and drug adaptation :

In the presence of renal insufficiency, many drugs require a change in dosage. This is most often necessary because the clearance of the drug is mainly renal, although it is also sometimes necessary because the drug is also nephrotoxic. In cases of pre-existing renal impairment, the drug should be used with caution. The first publication to study the value of cys C in this field looked at dose adjustment of digoxin in elderly subjects. It concluded that this new parameter was not superior to creatinine in predicting clearance of the drug. Other studies based on population pharmacokinetic methodology have definitively demonstrated the value of cys C in predicting the clearance of drugs eliminated exclusively or even partially by the kidneys, namely two cytotoxic drugs, topotecan and carboplatin (159).

2.5.6.1.5. Cys C and cardiovascular risks :

ESRD or stage 3 of the KDOQI classification is currently recognised as an independent risk factor for cardiovascular disease. The discovery of a biological marker of impaired renal function that is potentially earlier and less dependent on extra-renal factors than creatinine has prompted several teams, notably Shlipak (172), to study the relationship between cardiovascular disease, mortality and circulating cys-C levels. Epidemiological studies based on large cohorts of patients have clearly identified high levels of cys-C (above 1.30 mg/L) as an independent risk factor for cardiovascular disease. These values may be associated with cardiac morphological abnormalities, such as left ventricular hypertrophy or left ventricular dysfunction identified by ultrasound, functional abnormalities such as heart failure or exercise intolerance (173).

Consequently, Cys C appears to be an independent risk marker for cardiovascular disease with multifactorial potential (159).

2.5.6.2. Beta 2 microglobulin

ß2-M was discovered in 1968 by Berggard *et al.* in the urine of patients suffering from Wilson's disease or chronic cadmium poisoning. It is a globular protein similar *to* the light chain of the histocompatibility antigen of the *HLA* (human leucocyte antigens) system, which enables recognition between individuals and plays an important role in cell-cell relationships, with a decisive influence on grafts and transplants. ß2-M is present in many biological fluids, including blood and urine, but also in low concentrations in seminal, synovial, peritoneal, pleural and cerebrospinal fluids. ß2-M is a small globulin with a relative molar mass of 11.8 kDa(14).

It belongs to the group of "low molecular weight proteins" (*LMWP*) (100 amino acids). It is produced by all the body's nucleated cells (except the trophoblast), T lymphocytes, B lymphocytes and tumour cells when they are present. In humans, it is encoded by a gene located on chromosome 15. It exists in two forms, the free form in biological fluids and the form bound to the membranes of nucleated cells, where it forms the light chain of HLA class I molecules. It is filtered in the kidneys by the glomeruli, then reabsorbed and catabolised at tubular level. In the absence of renal impairment, the increase in plasma concentrations corresponds to an increase in synthesis (14).

2.5.6.2.1. Dosage technique

Depending on the assay technique, the test is carried out on serum or plasma. The young person does not appear to be essential. Haemolysis and hyperlipidaemia may interfere with the assay. For storage and transport, serum samples should be kept at +2 to +8°C for 8 days, or frozen within 24 hours of collection (174).

There are various methods for measuring ß2-M. The reference technique is a RIA (radioimmunoassay) test, which is long, expensive and subject to radiation protection regulations requiring suitable premises and qualified personnel. This technique is therefore not accessible to all laboratories. Studies on the analytical performance of an immuno-chemiluminescence technique and an immuno-turbidimetry technique on serum compared with that of RIA have shown that they are correlated, on dry tube and on heparinised tube, for the two non-isotopic techniques (174, 175).

2.5.6.2.2. Reference values and physio-pathological variations

In adults, serum β2-M is stable, with usual values of between 1.1 and 2.4 mg/l.

Newborns have higher levels than adults, while children up to puberty have lower levels. Serum levels increase after the age of 60. During pregnancy, serum ß2-M levels are higher (174).

Elevated serum concentrations of ß2-M are found in two distinct situations.

- **Increased synthesis:** observed in lymphoid proliferative diseases: multiple myeloma (MM), lymphomas, chronic lymphocytic leukaemia (CLL) and myelodysplastic syndromes (MDS). But also in inflammatory diseases, autoimmune diseases and CMV or HIV viral infections.
- **Decreased renal clearance**: observed in renal failure, there is a good correlation between serum β2- M concentration and glomerular filtration rate (14).

2.5.6.2.3. ß2-M and renal impairment

Numerous studies to date have demonstrated significant correlations between measures of renal function and serum ß2-M levels. These studies provide convincing reasons why renal filtration can be estimated using a ß2-M estimating equation (174).

The CKD-EPI group developed a GFR estimation equation based on ß2-M in a cohort of 2,380 patients, mainly Caucasians and African-Americans, with mean GFR (mGFR) measured serum creatinine and serum ß2-M levels of 47.5 (21.7) ml/min/1.73 m^2 , 1.9 (0.9) mg/dl and 4.3 (2.4) mg/l, respectively (39). ß2-M was highly positively correlated with cys-C and serum creatinine, with Pearson coefficients of 0.9 and 0.78, respectively (14).

Serum ß2-M was found to be inversely correlated with GFR with a Pearson value of 0.85. The authors used the least error regression model for equation development and included age, sex and race variables. Coefficients for β2-M were significant although small, similar to those for cys C, and smaller than those for creatinine (14).

In this cohort, the CKD-EPI ß2-M equation outperformed the CKD-EPI creatinine, cys C equations in terms of accuracy. Nevertheless, the CKD-EPI ß2- M equation has an advantage over the other CKD-EPI equations in that it is not affected by race, age or sex (14).

Only ethnicity (lower in blacks), smoking (higher in smokers) and proteinuria (higher in patients with proteinuria) were directly implicated in the elevation of ß2-M levels in multivariate adjusted models (175).

This disparity should be taken as evidence that ß2-M is a slightly superior marker of renal filtration, with stronger correlations with measured GFR and weaker correlations with non-renal factors such as creatinine(176).

However, the effects of non-renal determinants on other parameters affecting ß2-M kinetics negate this apparent advantage, so that the overall performance of the CKD-EPI ß2-M equation is comparable to that of other equations for estimating glomerular filtration rate (14).

> **Paediatric population**

Creatinine clearance is known to be an unreliable marker for measuring GFR in children, due to muscle mass. This is why other markers, including ß2-M, which is not influenced by muscle mass, have been studied. Furthermore, the recently developed formula CKD-Epi- Trace-ß2-M cannot be applied to children (176).

In summary, the use of serum ß2-M as a measure of glomerular filtration function does not appear to be as useful in children as in adults (177).

However, urinary excretion of ß2-M has been used in the diagnosis of a wide variety of renal diseases in children (14) .

> **Interest of ß2-M in tubular function**

Elimination of ß2-M from serum is mainly by glomerular filtration, but more than 99.9% of the filtered proteins are reabsorbed and catabolised in the proximal tubule, resulting in a minimal urinary concentration of ß2-M (generally less than 360 µg/l)

(14).

Tubular handling of ß2-M matures during the neonatal period. Urinary ß2-M excretion peaks on the fifth day of life and gradually decreases to adult levels at 3 months of age. This feature suggests that urinary ß2-M may not only be a reliable biomarker of tubular toxicity, but may even have an age-dependent performance (14).

A recent animal toxicology study evaluated the performance of neutrophil gelatinase-associated lipocalin (NGAL) and four urinary biomarkers deemed acceptable by regulatory authorities to detect acute drug-induced renal toxicity: ß2-M, cys C, kidney injury molecule-1 (KIM-1) and clusterin. In this particular study, urinary β2-\-1 and urinary cys C levels increased early (before histological changes were detected) and returned to the control range in the recovery phase. Furthermore, changes in plasma β2-\--1 paralleled changes in urinary β2-\-1. However, correlations between biomarker values varied according to the type of nephrotoxicity (175).

> ß2-M and renal transplantation

The identification of urinary biomarkers capable of detecting early tubular damage would be beneficial in helping to identify patients who require allograft biopsy, in order to prevent progression to chronic damage. These data are identical to those available in non-transplant CKD patients, GFR based on serum β2-\-1 (<30 vs. >60 ml/min) has been found to predict CV (cardiovascular ,overall mortality and dialysis renal failure in allograft recipients (158).

The predictive ability of elevations in serum β2-\-1 for subsequent allograft loss has also been reported by other groups (174).

2.5.6.2.4. β2-M and haemato-oncological pathology

In haematological malignancies such as leukaemia, lymphoma and multiple myeloma, serum β2-\-1 is elevated despite preserved renal function. It has been reported that 60% of patients with mantle cell lymphoma have elevated serum β2-\-1 prior to treatment. This elevated value is independently associated with the poor prognosis of most haematological malignancies (178).

These associations persist despite adjustment for well-validated clinical prognostic scores and therapeutic indicators. In multiple myeloma, serum ß2-M levels are the main determinant of the International Staging System (ISS). ß2-M predicts not only prognosis but also progression of asymptomatic disease and even outcome after stem cell transplantation (78).

2.5.6.2.5. *ß2-M* and autoimmune diseases

Serum levels of β2-M are also elevated in autoimmune diseases. Very high serum levels are seen in patients with systemic lupus erythematosus and adult Still's disease, particularly in those with active disease and haemophagocytic syndrome. Following treatment, serum β2-\--1 levels decrease significantly. Urinary β2-M correlates with global and renal activity scores and proteinuria (179).

2.5.6.3. Other plasma and urine biomarkers

Biomarkers of glomerular damage, tubular damage, inflammation and oxidative stress precede albuminuria in some patients and may therefore be useful for early prediction of ND, although most of them have yet to be validated (180, 181).

Table 15: Summary of certain new biomarkers for diabetic nephropathy (199)

Biomarker	Type of renal injury	TIDM	T2DM	Pre-microalbuminuria^	Predicts microalbuminuria
Urinary transferrin	Glomerular injury	+	+	+	+
Urinary TNF-a	Glomerular injury	+	+	+	+
Urinary type IV collagen	Glomerular/tubular injury	+	+	+	+
Urinary fibronectin	Glomerular injury	+	+		
Urinary GAGs	Glomerular injury	+	+	+	
Urinary NAG	Tubular injury	+	+	+	+
Urinary L-PGDS	Glomerular injury		+	+	+

Note: ^Appears in urine before microalbuminuria.

Abbreviations: TIDM, type I diabetes mellitus; T2DM, type 2 diabetes mellitus; TNF-", tumor necrosis factor ": GAGs, glycosaminoglycans; NAG, N-acetyl-ß-D- glucosaminidase; L-PGDS. lipocalin-type prostaglandin D synthase.

2.5.6.3.1. Tubulointerstitial biomarkers

A large number of ND biomarkers have been identified by transcriptomic and proteomic analyses of kidney tissue after injury. There is therefore a bias in favour of the identification of renal tubulointerstitial markers, reflecting their greater mass compared with the vascular and glomerular compartments (182).

Biomarkers such as cys C, KIM-1, NGAL, angiotensinogen, periostin and monocyte chemoattractant protein-1 (MCP-1) reflect tubular damage (183).

Tubular markers of kidney damage may be able to reflect the degree of kidney damage in diabetic patients.

Urinary liver-type fatty acid-binding protein (L-FABP), NGAL and KIM-1 are newly established tubular biomarkers that have been reported as early detectors of acute kidney injury.

- Renal proximal tubular cells abundantly express L- FABP and urinary excretion of this molecule is high in diabetics even before the development of glomerular lesions or albuminuria.
- NGAL is also considered to be a sensitive and more accurate early predictor of acute kidney injuryê. Higher levels of urinary NGAL have been associated with lower GFR in T2DM with macro albuminuria (184-186).
- KIM-1 is a membrane protein expressed on the apical membrane of proximal renal tubule cells and reflects tubular damage in the most advanced stages of renal disease in diabetic patients.

Urinary levels of these tubular markers during the progression of DN reflect not only the severity of renal injury but also the degree of tubulointerstitial fibrosis. In contrast to the markers mentioned above, angiotensin-converting enzyme 2 (ACE2), a homologue of ACE, appears to play a protective role in diabetic kidney disease and is an important determinant of ND (186, 187).

2.5.6.3.2. Glomerular biomarkers

These biomarkers include transferrin, immunoglobulin

G (IgG), ceruleoplasmin, type IV collagen, laminin, glycosaminoglycans (GAGs), prostaglandin D synthase-type lipocalin (L-PGDS), fibronectin, podocyte-podocalyxin and VEGF (vascular endothelial growth factor) (180).

Interestingly, new approaches can be used to identify potential new biomarkers for ND.

In terms of glomerular biomarkers, it has been shown that urinary transferrin is a more reliable marker of the glomerulus than albuminuria. Some reports indicate that prior to the development of microalbuminuria, urinary transferrin appears to be higher in diabetic subjects than in their healthy controls. The albumin/transferrin ratio is significantly lower in diabetic patients with normo albuminuria and microalbuminuria than in those with macro albuminuria (188). Furthermore, urinary transferrin predicts the development of microalbuminuria in T2DM patients with normo albuminuria. In diabetic patients with macroalbuminuria, urinary transferrin excretion is positively correlated with EUA. However, transferrinuria is also observed in primary glomerulonephritis, as well as certain systemic diseases that secondarily affect the glomerulus, thus highlighting its lack of specificity for ND (181).

Urinary IgG is another related biomarker. Immunoglobulin G is an anionic plasma protein that crosses the glomerulus with difficulty, but appears in the urine concomitantly with urinary transferrin, urinary ceruloplasmin and urinary orosomucoid before the onset of microalbuminuria, suggesting the ability of increased urinary IgG elimination to predict the onset of microalbuminuria in DM patients (189).

Laminin and type IV collagen are components of the glomerular basement membrane, although the latter is also a component of the mesangial matrix. Given that elevated urinary levels of type IV collagen are observed in normo albuminurics with T1DM, this biomarker has even been considered as a specific indicator of early DN (190).

In addition, some studies indicate that urinary excretion of type IV collagen in T2DM is related to UAE, while other investigators have shown that T2DM patients with evidence of renal disease have a significantly higher type IV collagen/albumin ratio than their non-diabetic counterparts with nephropathy (191).

These results support the possible use of urinary type IV collagen in the differentiation of DN and non-diabetic nephropathy.

Finally, urinary type IV collagen has also been shown to be more sensitive than albuminuria in detecting renal damage in patients with T2DM, although other authors have reported that a third of patients with microalbuminuria do not have increased urinary excretion of type IV collagen(192).

Urinary fibronectin is probably another useful biomarker of DN, but its relevance in relation to albuminuria needs to be validated by other studies.

Urinary GAGs are increased in ND patients with normo albuminuria and are associated with other tubular markers such as Tamm-Horsfall protein, which expresses distal tubular dysfunction in ND patients. GAGs are also present in the tubular basement membrane (193).

Finally, L-PGDS is a biomarker associated with damage to glomerular capillary walls and reflects their increased permeability. Although it is essentially considered to be predictive of kidney damage, it is less relevant as an early biomarker of ND (181, 187).

2.5.6.3.3. Biomarker of renal inflammation

During ND, renal inflammation and the influx of inflammatory cells cause the release of interleukins and cytokines, such as TNF- α, MCP-1, TGF-ß1, IL-1ß, IL-6 and IL-8, creating a pro-inflammatory microenvironment that amplifies damage. Several studies have examined their potential clinical use in the assessment of ND (194).

Other biomarkers of inflammation, which are also glomerular markers, are IL-18, interferon gamma induce protein (IP-10), monocyte chemoattractant protein1 (MCP-1), granulocyte colony-stimulating factor (G-CSF), eotaxins, RANTES (regulated on activation, normal T cell expressed and secreted) or CCL-5, and orosomucoid.

S Il-18 is a pro-inflammatory cytokine derived from mononuclear cells, and its serum and urine levels have been reported to correlate positively with albumin, while its serum levels correlate positively with carotid intima-media thickness in patients with T2DM, and may therefore be a predictor of progression of DN, as well as cardiovascular disease (195).

S IP-10 and MCP-1 are other pro-inflammatory cytokines whose serum levels are significantly increased in subjects with T2DM.

S Serum and urinary G-CSF levels are also increased in the early stages of ND, while urinary excretion rates of RANTES (or CCL-5) and eotaxin have been noted to be significantly higher in patients with hyperfiltration than in T1DM patients with normo filtration (194).

S Like RANTES, which is a chemotactic cytokine, eotaxin is a subfamily of eosinophil chemotactic cytokines, composed of eotaxin-1 and eotaxin-2.Elevated urinary levels of eotaxin and RANTES, arising from hyperfiltration in the diabetic kidney, result from elevated intraglomerular pressure which causes renal inflammation (196).

2.5.6.3.4. Biomarkers of oxidative stress

A typical example of an oxidative stress biomarker is urinary 8-oxo-7,8-dihydro-2-deoxyguanosine (8oHdG).

This marker is produced as a result of oxidative DNA damage and appears in the urine without being metabolised. Remarkably, urinary 8oHdG has been reported to be a useful clinical marker for predicting the development of Creutzfeldt-Jakob disease according to the WHO definition (197).

Higher levels of 8-oHdG in the urine indicate significant disease progression compared with low or moderate levels (196).

2.5.6.3.5. Emerging biomarkers

> MicroRNAs (miRNAs)

These are attractive new diagnostic biomarkers for MND.

They are small endogenous non-coding RNAs (20-30 nucleotides) that regulate gene expression by binding to the 3' untranslated regions of specific mRNAs, inducing their degradation or translational repression. miRNAs have therefore been implicated in the post-transcriptional regulation of gene expression and the control of various processes such as apoptosis, DNA repair, the response to oxidative stress, cancer and cell development (198).

> Long non-coding RNA

Long non-coding RNAs (lncRNAs) are non-coding transcripts of variable size (ranging from 200 nucleotides to 100 kbp) with no protein-coding function. It has been found that lncRNA expression correlates with miRNA expression in ND models (199). Several studies have implicated a role for plasmacytoma translocation variant 1 (PVT1) in the pathogenesis of ND (15).

> Urinary exosomes

Urinary exosomes are small vesicles (40-100 nm) released by most kidney cells. They harbour various types of cytosolic, membrane and transport proteins, as well as nucleic acids (200). Exosomes reflect the pathophysiological status of their host cells and have emerged as a promising non-invasive source of biomarkers for DN and as an indicator of disease stage and progression (15).

> Microparticles

Microparticles (MPs) are extracellular vesicles released from the cell surface in the event of stress or damage. MPs are larger than exosomes (0.1-1 μm) and have a particular molecular composition. In other words, they expose phosphatidylserine at the surface. MPs are released from kidney cells in the event of glycaemic disturbance and can be detected in plasma and urine before the onset of ND (15, 198).

References

1. Diabetes A. Canadian Diabetes Association 2008 Clinical Practice Guidelines for the Prevention and Management of Diabetes in Canada. Can J Diabetes. 2008;32:S1-S225.

2. diabete Fid. IDF diabete atlas 2019.

3. Tenenbaum M, Bonnefond A, Froguel P, Abderrahmani A. Physiopathology of the diabetes. Revue Francophone des Laboratoires. 2018;2018(502):26-32.

4. Vionnet AC, Jornayvaz FR. Classification of diabetes: towards increasing heterogeneity. Rev Med Suisse. 2015;11:1234-7.

5. SCHEEN A, Paquot N. Le diabete de type 2: voyage au coeur d'une maladie complexe. Revue Médicale de Liège. 2012;67(5-6).

6. Schlienger J-L. Complications of type 2 diabetes. La Presse Médicale. 2013;42(5):839-48.

7. Fonfrède M. Diabète et rein. Revue Francophone des Laboratoires. 2013;2013(455):45-50.

8. Roussel R. Natural history of diabetic nephropathy. Metabolic diseases medicine. 2011;5:S8-S13.

9. Avinash S, Singh V, Agarwal A, Chatterjee S, Araya V. Identification and Stratification of Diabetic Kidney Disease Using Serum Cystatin C and Serum Creatinine Based Estimating Equations in Type 2 Diabetes: A Comparative Analysis. The Journal of the Association of Physicians of India. 2015;63(11):28-35.

10. Rigalleau V, Beauvieux MC, Gonzalez C, Raffaitin C, Lasseur C, Combe C, et al. Estimation of renal function in patients with diabetes. Diabetes Metab. 2011;37(5):359- 66. Epub 2011/06/18.

11. Rigalleau V, Beauvieux MC, Gonzalez C, Raffaitin C, Lasseur C, Combe C, et al. Estimation of renal function in patients with diabetes. Diabetes & Metabolism. 2011;37(5):359-66.

12. Tziomalos K, Athyros VG. Diabetic nephropathy: new risk factors and improvements in diagnosis. The review of diabetic studies: RDS. 2015;12(1-2):110.

13. Pelaez A, Dinic M, Roche F, Barthélémy J, Alamartine E, Cavalier E, et al. Cystatin C, inflammation and autonomic dysfunction: a hidden "ménage à trois"? Nephrology & Therapeutics. 2020;16(5):310-1.

14. Argyropoulos CP, Chen SS, Ng Y-H, Roumelioti M-E, Shaffi K, Singh PP, et al. Rediscovering beta-2 microglobulin as a biomarker across the spectrum of kidney diseases. Frontiers in medicine. 2017;4:73.

15. Campion CG, Sanchez-Ferras O, Batchu SN. Potential role of serum and urinary biomarkers in diagnosis and prognosis of diabetic nephropathy. Canadian journal of kidney health and disease. 2017;4:2054358117705371.

16. Krzesinski J-M, Scheen A. Diabetic kidney disease: current management and

future prospects. Swiss Medical Journal. 2015;11(483):1534-8.
17. ADA E. Diagnosis and classification of diabetes mellitus new criteria. Diabetes & Metabolism (Paris). 1999;25:72-83.
18. Federation ID. IDF Diabetes Atlas 9 eme edition 2019 2019.
19. Gariani K, Tran C, Philippe J. Glycated haemoglobin. Rev Med Suisse. 2011;7:1238- 42.
20. Baynes HW. Classification, pathophysiology, diagnosis and management of diabetes mellitus. J diabetes metab. 2015;6(5):1-9.
21. Organization WH. Classification of diabetes mellitus. 2019.
22. BIOLOGICAL CRITERIA D, SUGAR D. Definition and classification of diabetes. Médecine Nucléaire-Imagerie fonctionnelle et métabolique. 2001;25(2):91.
23. Chevenne D, Fonfrède M. Actualités en diabétologie. Immunoanalysis & Specialised Biology. 2007;22(2):95-100.
24. Chevenne D, Fonfrède M. Actualités en diabétologie. Immunoanalysis & Specialised Biology. 2007;22(2):95-100.
25. Spinas G, Lehmann R, editors. Diabetes mellitus: Diagnosis, classification and pathogenesis, Rev. Forum Med; 2001.
26. World Health O. Global Diabetes Report. 2016.
27. Dinar Y, Belahsen R. Diabetes Mellitus in Morocco: Situation and Challenges of Diabetes Care. Journal of Scientific Research and Reports. 2014:2477-85.
28. Ahmed Chetoui KK, El Kardoudi A, Boutahar K, Chigr F, Najimi M. Epidemiology of diabetes in Morocco: review of data, analysis and perspectives. Int J Scientific Eng Res. 2018;9:1310-6.
29. Zaoui S, Biémont C, Meguenni K. Epidemiological approach to diabetes in urban and rural settings in the Tlemcen region (western Algeria). Cahiers d'études et de recherches francophones/Santé. 2007;17(1):15-21.
30. MOSSI KE, BALAKA A, TCHAMDJA T, DJAGADOU KA, Sama HD, APETI S, et al. Prevalence of complications of diabetes mellitus at the Clinique médico-chirurgicale du CHU Sylvanus Olympio de Lomé. Revue Africaine de Médecine Interne. 2019;6(1-3):42-8.
31. Orban J-C, Ichai C. Acute metabolic complications of diabetes. Réanimation. 2008;17(8):761-7.
32. Tenoutasse S, Mouraux T, Dorchy H. Diabetic ketoacidosis: diagnosis, management and prevention. Rev Med Brux. 2010;31:71-6.
33. Orban JC, Ghaddab A, Chatti O, Ichai C. Lactic acidosis and metformin. Annales Françaises d'Anesthésie et de Réanimation. 2006;25(10):1046-52.
34. Salpeter SR, Greyber E, Pasternak GA, Salpeter EE. Risk of fatal and non-fatal lactic acidosis with metformin use in type 2 diabetes mellitus: systematic review and metaanalysis. Archives of internal medicine. 2003;163(21):2594-602.
35. Ardigo S, Philippe J. Hypoglycaemia and diabetes. Rev Med Suisse. 2008;4:1376-

82.
36. Deshpande AD, Harris-Hayes M, Schootman M. Epidemiology of diabetes and diabetes-related complications. Physical therapy. 2008;88(11):1254-64.
37. Constantino MI, Molyneaux L, Limacher-Gisler F, Al-Saeed A, Luo C, Wu T, et al. Long-term complications and mortality in young-onset diabetes: type 2 diabetes is more hazardous and lethal than type 1 diabetes. Diabetes care. 2013;36(12):3863-9.
38. Said G. Diabetic neuropathies. Neurologie com. 2009;1(2):40-4.
39. diabete acd. Canadian Diabetes Association 2008 Clinical Practice Guidelines for the Prevention and Treatment of Diabetes. Canadian Journals of Diabetes. 2008;32:225.
40. Flagothier C, Quatresooz P, Bourguignon R, Pierard C, Pierard G. Cutaneous stigmata of diabetes. Revue Médicale de Liège. 2005;60(5-6):553-9.
41. Malek R. Diabetes mellitus and COVID-19 Diabetes mellitus and COVID-19.
42. Paquot N, Radermecker R. Covid-19 and diabetes. Revue Medicale de Liege. 2020;75:138-45.
43. Hartmann-Boyce J, Morris E, Goyder C, Kinton J, Perring J, Nunan D, et al. Diabetes and COVID-19: risks, management, and learnings from other national disasters. Diabetes Care. 2020;43(8):1695-703.
44. SCHEEN A, Paquot N. Le diabete de type 2: voyage au coeur d'une maladie complexe. Revue Médicale de Liège. 2012;67(5-6):326-31.
45. Fery F, Paquot N. Etiopathogenesis and pathophysiology of type 2 diabetes. Revue Médicale de Liège. 2005;60(5-6):361-8.
46. Druet C, Bourdel-Marchasson I, Weill A, Eschwege E, Penfornis A, Fosse S, et al. Type 2 diabetes in France: epidemiology, changes in the quality of care, social and economic burden. Entred 2007. La Presse Médicale. 2013;42(5):830-8.
47. Alberti KGMM, Zimmet P, Shaw J. International Diabetes Federation: a consensus on Type 2 diabetes prevention. Diabetic Medicine. 2007;24(5):451-63.
48. Atlas D. International diabetes federation. IDF Diabetes Atlas, 7th edn Brussels, Belgium: International Diabetes Federation. 2015.
49. Chatterjee S, Khunti K, Davies MJ. Type 2 diabetes. The Lancet. 2017;389(10085):2239-51.
50. Elbein SC, Wegner K, Kahn SE. Reduced beta-cell compensation to the insulin resistance associated with obesity in members of caucasian familial type 2 diabetic kindreds. Diabetes care. 2000;23(2):221-7.
51. Matthews DR, Hosker J, Rudenski A, Naylor B, Treacher D, Turner R. Homeostasis model assessment: insulin resistance and β-cell function from fasting plasma glucose and insulin concentrations in man. Diabetologia. 1985;28(7):412-9.
52. Guillausseau P-J, Laloi-Michelin M. Physiopathology of type 2 diabetes. La revue de médecine interne. 2003;24(11):730-7.
53. Rigalleau V, Lang J, Gin H. Etiology and pathophysiology of type 2 diabetes.

Endocrinologie-Nutrition. 2007;10:10-366.
54. Lindsay J, McKillop A, Mooney M, O'Harte F, Bell P, Flatt P. Demonstration of increased concentrations of circulating glycated insulin in human Type 2 diabetes using a novel and specific radioimmunoassay. Diabetologia. 2003;46(4):475-8.
55. White MF. IRS proteins and the common path to diabetes. American Journal of Physiology-Endocrinology And Metabolism. 2002;283(3):E413-E22.
56. Prentki M, Nolan CJ. Islet β cell failure in type 2 diabetes. The Journal of clinical investigation. 2006;116(7):1802-12.
57. Bouche C, Serdy S, Kahn CR, Goldfine AB. The cellular fate of glucose and its relevance in type 2 diabetes. Endocrine reviews. 2004;25(5):807-30.
58. Eguchi K, Nagai R. Islet inflammation in type 2 diabetes and physiology. The Journal of clinical investigation. 2017;127(1):14-23.
59. Rissanen A, Howard C, Botha J, Thuren T, Investigators G. Effect of anti-IL-1ß antibody (canakinumab) on insulin secretion rates in impaired glucose tolerance or type 2 diabetes: results of a randomized, placebo-controlled trial. Diabetes, Obesity and Metabolism. 2012;14(12):1088-96.
60. Richardson S, Willcox A, Bone A, Foulis A, Morgan N. Islet-associated macrophages in type 2 diabetes. Diabetologia. 2009;52(8):1686-8.
61. Rorive M, Letiexhe M, Scheen A, Ziegler O. Obesity and type 2 diabetes. Revue médicale de liège. 2005;60(5-6):374-82.
62. Fumeron F. From obesity to type 2 diabetes: epidemiology and pathophysiology. Sci Food. 2005;25(5-6):339-47.
63. Dembélé M, Sidibe A, Traoré H, Tchombou H, Zounet B, Traore A, et al. Association HTA-Diabète sucré dans le service de Médecine Interne de l'Hopital du Point G-Bamako. Médecine d'Afrique noire. 2000;47:276-80.
64. Monabeka H, Bouenizabila E, Mupangu M, KIBANGOU N, ETITIELE F. Hypertension and diabetes mellitus in 152 hypertensive diabetics. Médecine d'Afrique Noire. 1998;45(2):105-9.
65. Krzesinski J-M, Weekers L. Hypertension and diabetes. Revue medicale de Liege. 2005;60(5-6, May-Jun):572-7.
66. Vergès B. Pathophysiology of dyslipidaemia in type 2 diabetes: new perspectives. Medicine of Metabolic Diseases. 2019;13(2):140-6.
67. Tanguy B, Aboyans V. Dyslipidemia and diabetes. Revues Générales Métabolisme. 2014:37-41.
68. Nilsson PM, Gudbjörnsdottir S, Eliasson B, Cederholm J. Smoking is associated with increased HbA1c values and microalbuminuria in patients with diabetes - data from the National Diabetes Register in Sweden. Diabetes & Metabolism. 2004;30(3):261-8.
69. Smith U. Smoking elicits the insulin resistance syndrome: new aspects of the harmful effect of smoking. Wiley Online Library; 1995. p. 435-7.

70. Magis D, Geronooz I, Scheen A. Smoking, insulin resistance and type 2 diabetes. Revue Médicale de Liège. 2002;57(9):575-81.
71. Eliasson B, Attvall S, Taskinen M-R, Smith U. The insulin resistance syndrome in smokers is related to smoking habits. Arteriosclerosis and thrombosis: a journal of vascular biology. 1994;14(12):1946-50.
72. Duclos M, Sanz C, Gautier J-F. Physical activity and prevention of type 2 diabetes. Metabolic diseases medicine. 2010;4(2):147-51.
73. Lameira D, Lejeune S, Mourad J-J, editors. Metabolic syndrome: its epidemiology and risks. Annales de Dermatologie et de Vénéréologie; 2008: Elsevier. 74. Ford ES, Giles WH, Dietz WH. Prevalence of the metabolic syndrome among US adults: findings from the third National Health and Nutrition Examination Survey. Jama. 2002;287(3):356-9.
75. Scheen A. The metabolic syndrome: pathophysiology and treatment. Atherosclerosis, atherothrombosis. 2006:162-90.
76. Junien C, Gallou-Kabani C, Vigé A, Gross M-S. Nutritional epigenomics of metabolic syndrome. M/S: médecine sciences. 2005;21(4):396-404.
77. Scheen A, Van Gaal L. Le diabete de type 2 au coeur du syndrome metabolique: plaidoyer pour une prise en charge globale. Revue Médicale de Liège. 2005;60(5-6):566- 71.
78. Remuzzi G, Benigni A, Remuzzi A. Mechanisms of progression and regression of renal lesions of chronic nephropathies and diabetes. The Journal of clinical investigation. 2006;116(2):288-96.
79. López-Novoa JM, Rodríguez-Peña AB, Ortiz A, Martínez-Salgado C, López Hernández FJ. Etiopathology of chronic tubular, glomerular and renovascular nephropathies: Clinical implications. Journal of Translational Medicine. 2011;9(1):13.
80. Adler AI, Stevens RJ, Manley SE, Bilous RW, Cull CA, Holman RR, et al. Development and progression of nephropathy in type 2 diabetes: the United Kingdom Prospective Diabetes Study (UKPDS 64). Kidney international. 2003;63(1):225-32.
81. Dordevic G, Racki S. Bozidar Vujicic, Tamara Turk, Zeljka Crncevic-Orlic. Pathophysiology and Complications of Diabetes Mellitus. 2012:71.
82. Tonelli M, Muntner P, Lloyd A, Manns BJ, Klarenbach S, Pannu N, et al. Risk of coronary events in people with chronic kidney disease compared with those with diabetes: a population-level cohort study. The Lancet. 2012;380(9844):807-14.
83. Dabla PK. Renal function in diabetic nephropathy. World journal of diabetes. 2010;1(2):48-56.
84. Mogensen C. Microalbuminuria predicts clinical proteinuria and early mortality in maturity-onset diabetes. New England journal of medicine. 1984;310(6):356-60.
85. Afkarian M, Sachs MC, Kestenbaum B, Hirsch IB, Tuttle KR, Himmelfarb J, et al. Kidney disease and increased mortality risk in type 2 diabetes. Journal of the

American Society of Nephrology. 2013;24(2):302-8.
86. FAGOT CAMPAGNA A, Fosse S, POUTIGNAT N, WEILL A, PAUMIER A. Characteristics, vascular risk and complications in diabetics in metropolitan France: major changes between Entred 2001 and Entred 2007. Bulletin épidémiologique hebdomadaire. 2009(42-43):450-5.
87. Villar E. Diabetes-related kidney disease: epidemiology and costs. Medicine of Metabolic Diseases. 2011;5:S2-S7.
88. Barsoum RS. Burden of chronic kidney disease: North Africa. Kidney international supplements. 2013;3(2):164-6.
89. NIBOUCHE-HATTAB WN. ETUDE DE LA MORBIDITE AU MOMENT DU DIAGNOSTIC DU DIABETE DE TYPE 2 DE L'ADULTE: Université D'Alger 1; 2015.
90. Weekers L, Krzesinski J-M. Diabetic nephropathy. Revue Médicale de Liège. 2005;60(5-6, May-Jun):479-86.
91. Dabla PK. Renal function in diabetic nephropathy. World journal of diabetes. 2010;1(2):48.
92. Schena FP, Gesualdo L. Pathogenetic mechanisms of diabetic nephropathy. Journal of the American society of nephrology. 2005;16(3 suppl 1):S30-S3.
93. Reach G, Altman J, Slama G, Tchohroutsky G. Causes and mechanisms of diabetic microangiopathy and neuropathy. The "glucose hypothesis" and its consequences. Vascular complications of diabetes (Eds Tchobroutsky G, Slama G, Assan R, Freychet P), Pradel, Paris. 1994:53-62.
94. Wolf G. Molecular mechanisms of diabetic kidney disease. Actualités néphrologiques Jean Hamburger. 2005:205-16.
95. Gariani K, de Seigneux S, Pechère-Bertschi A, Philippe J, Martin P-Y. Diabetic nephropathy. Swiss Medical Journal. 2012(330):473.
96. Dronavalli S, Duka I, Bakris GL. The pathogenesis of diabetic nephropathy. Nature clinical practice Endocrinology & metabolism. 2008;4(8):444-52.
97. Pantsulaia T. Role of TGF-beta in pathogenesis of diabetic nephropathy. Georgian medical news. 2006(131):13-8.
98. Chalkia A, Gakiopoulou H, Theohari I, Foukas PG, Vassilopoulos D, Petras D. Transforming Growth Factor-ß1/Smad Signaling in Glomerulonephritis and Its Association with Progression to Chronic Kidney Disease. American Journal of Nephrology. 2021;52(8):653-65.
99. Magee C, Grieve DJ, Watson CJ, Brazil DP. Diabetic nephropathy: a tangled web to unweave. Cardiovascular drugs and therapy. 2017;31(5):579-92.
100. Alicic RZ, Rooney MT, Tuttle KR. Diabetic kidney disease: challenges, progress, and possibilities. Clinical journal of the American Society of Nephrology. 2017;12(12):2032-45. 101. Ritz E. Clinical manifestations and natural history of diabetic kidney disease. Medical Clinics. 2013;97(1):19-29.
102. Satchell SC. The glomerular endothelium emerges as a key player in diabetic

nephropathy. Kidney international. 2012;82(9):949-51.
103. Oguntibeju O. Pathophysiology and Complications of Diabetes Mellitus: BoD - Books on Demand; 2012.
104. Pylypchuk G, Beaubien E. Diabetic nephropathy. Prevention and early referral. Canadian Family Physician. 2000;46(3):636-42.
105. Pugliese G. Updating the natural history of diabetic nephropathy. Acta diabetologica. 2014;51(6):905-15.
106. Tonna S, El-Osta A, Cooper ME, Tikellis C. Metabolic memory and diabetic nephropathy: potential role for epigenetic mechanisms. Nature Reviews Nephrology. 2010;6(6):332-41.
107. Levin A, Stevens PE, Bilous RW, Coresh J, De Francisco AL, De Jong PE, et al. Kidney Disease: Improving Global Outcomes (KDIGO) CKD Work Group. KDIGO 2012 clinical practice guideline for the evaluation and management of chronic kidney disease. Kidney international supplements. 2013;3(1):1-150.
108. Hovind P, Tarnow L, Rossing P, Graae M, Torp I, Binder C, et al. Predictors for the development of microalbuminuria and macroalbuminuria in patients with type 1 diabetes: inception cohort study. Bmj. 2004;328(7448):1105.
109. MacIsaac RJ, Tsalamandris C, Panagiotopoulos S, Smith TJ, McNeil KJ, Jerums G. Nonalbuminuric renal insufficiency in type 2 diabetes. Diabetes care. 2004;27(1):195-200.
110. Araki S-i, Haneda M, Sugimoto T, Isono M, Isshiki K, Kashiwagi A, et al. Factors associated with frequent remission of microalbuminuria in patients with type 2 diabetes. Diabetes. 2005;54(10):2983-7.
111. Tziomalos K, Athyros VG. Diabetic Nephropathy: New Risk Factors and Improvements in Diagnosis. The review of diabetic studies: RDS. 2015;12(1-2):110-8. Epub 2015/08/10.
112. Retnakaran R, Cull CA, Thorne KI, Adler AI, Holman RR, Group US. Risk factors for renal dysfunction in type 2 diabetes: UK Prospective Diabetes Study 74. diabetes. 2006;55(6):1832-9.
113. Bakris GL, Weir MR, Shanifar S, Zhang Z, Douglas J, van Dijk DJ, et al. Effects of blood pressure level on progression of diabetic nephropathy: results from the RENAAL study. Archives of internal medicine. 2003;163(13):1555-65.
114. Harper CR, Jacobson TA. Managing dyslipidemia in chronic kidney disease. Journal of the American College of Cardiology. 2008;51(25):2375-84.
115. Ejerblad E, Fored CM, Lindblad P, Fryzek J, McLaughlin JK, Nyrén O. Obesity and risk for chronic renal failure. Journal of the American society of nephrology. 2006;17(6):1695-702.
116. Kramer HJ, Nguyen QD, Curhan G, Hsu C-y. Renal insufficiency in the absence of albuminuria and retinopathy among adults with type 2 diabetes mellitus. Jama. 2003;289(24):3273-7.

117. Christensen PK, Larsen S, Horn T, Olsen S, Parving H-H. Causes of albuminuria in patients with type 2 diabetes without diabetic retinopathy. Kidney international. 2000;58(4):1719-31.
118. Chavers BM, Mauer SM, Ramsay RC, Steffes MW. Relationship between retinal and glomerular lesions in IDDM patients. Diabetes. 1994;43(3):441-6.
119. Retinopathy WESoD. III. Prevalence and risk of diabetic retinopathy when age at diagnosis is 30 or more years. Arch Ophthalmol. 1984;102:527-32.
120. Sandholm N, Salem RM, McKnight AJ, Brennan EP, Forsblom C, Isakova T, et al. New susceptibility loci associated with kidney disease in type 1 diabetes. 2012.
121. Hadjadj S, Weekers L, Marre M. Genetics of diabetic nephropathy. Sang Thrombose Vaisseaux. 2000;12(3).
122. Vlassara H. Recent progress in advanced glycation end products and diabetic complications. Diabetes. 1997;46(Supplement_2):S19-S25.
123. Heesom AE, Hibberd ML, Millward A, Demaine AG. Polymorphism in the 5'-end of the aldose reductase gene is strongly associated with the development of diabetic nephropathy in type I diabetes. Diabetes. 1997;46(2):287-91.
124. Hadjadj S, Weekers L, Marre M. Genetics of diabetic nephropathy. Sang Thrombose Vaisseaux. 2000;12(3):151-6.
125. Krolewski AS, Canessa M, Warram JH, Laffel LM, Christlieb R, Knowler WC, et al. Predisposition to hypertension and susceptibility to renal disease in insulin-dependent diabetes mellitus. New England Journal of Medicine. 1988;318(3):140-5.
126. Ng D, Tai B, Koh D, Tan K, Chia K. Angiotensin-I converting enzyme insertion/deletion polymorphism and its association with diabetic nephropathy: a metaanalysis of studies reported between 1994 and 2004 and comprising 14,727 subjects. Diabetologia. 2005;48(5):1008-16.
127. Rigalleau V, Gonzalez C, Combe C, Gin H. Kidney disease in T2DM: how to ensure diagnosis? Médecine des Maladies Métaboliques. 2011;5:S14-S8.
128. Tuttle KR, Bakris GL, Bilous RW, Chiang JL, de Boer IH, Goldstein-Fuchs J, et al. Diabetic kidney disease: a report from an ADA Consensus Conference. Diabetes Care. 2014;37(10):2864-83. Epub 2014/09/25.
129. Tuttle KR, Bakris GL, Bilous RW, Chiang JL, De Boer IH, Goldstein-Fuchs J, et al. Diabetic kidney disease: a report from an ADA Consensus Conference. American journal of kidney diseases. 2014;64(4):510-33.
130. Piccoli GB, Grassi G, Cabiddu G, Nazha M, Roggero S, Capizzi I, et al. Diabetic Kidney Disease: A Syndrome Rather Than a Single Disease. The review of diabetic studies: RDS. 2015;12(1-2):87-109. Epub 2015/08/10.
131. Nelson RG, Tuttle KR. The new KDOQITM clinical practice guidelines and clinical practice recommendations for diabetes and CKD. Blood purification. 2007;25(1):112-4.
132. Tuttle KR, Bakris GL, Bilous RW, Chiang JL, De Boer IH, Goldstein-Fuchs J, et al.

Diabetic kidney disease: a report from an ADA Consensus Conference. Diabetes care. 2014;37(10):2864-83.
133. MacIsaac RJ, Ekinci EI. Progression of diabetic kidney disease in the absence of albuminuria. Diabetes Care. 2019;42(10):1842-4.
134. Kramer H, Molitch ME. Screening for kidney disease in adults with diabetes. Diabetes Care. 2005;28(7):1813-6.
135. Livio F, Biollaz J, Burnier M. Estimation of renal function by the MDRD equation: interest and limitations for drug dose adjustment. Rev Med Suisse. 2008;4(181):2596-600.
136. Stevens LA, Coresh J, Feldman HI, Greene T, Lash JP, Nelson RG, et al. Evaluation of the modification of diet in renal disease study equation in a large diverse population. Journal of the American Society of Nephrology. 2007;18(10):2749-57.
137. Prigent A, editor. Monitoring renal function and limitations of renal function tests. Seminars in nuclear medicine; 2008: Elsevier.
138. Meier P. Markers of renal function and their predictive values. Caduseus Express. 2009;11(9).
139. Maillard N, Delanaye P, Mariat C. Investigation of renal glomerular function: estimation of glomerular filtration rate. Nephrology & Therapeutics. 2015;11(1):54-67.
140. Dussol B. Méthodes d'exploration de la fonction rénale: intérêt et limites des formules permettant d'estimer la fonction rénale. Immuno-analysis & Specialised Biology. 2011;26(1):6-12.
141. Levey AS, Bosch JP, Lewis JB, Greene T, Rogers N, Roth D, et al. A more accurate method to estimate glomerular filtration rate from serum creatinine: a new prediction equation. Annals of internal medicine. 1999;130(6):461-70.
142. Piéroni L, Delanaye P, Boutten A, Bargnoux A-S, Rozet E, Delatour V, et al. A multicentric evaluation of IDMS-traceable creatinine enzyme assays. Clinica Chimica Acta. 2011;412(23-24):2070-5.
143. Froissart M, Delanaye P, Seronie-Vivien S, Cristol J-P, editors. Evaluation of renal function: an update. Annales de Biologie Clinique; 2008: John Libbey Eurotext.
144. Dussol B. Méthodes d'exploration de la fonction rénale : intérêt et limites des formules permettant d'estimer la fonction rénale. Immuno-analysis & Specialised Biology. 2011;26(1):6-12.
145. Roger C, Carlier M-C. Albuminuria, microalbuminuria and diabetes. Revue Francophone des Laboratoires. 2018;2018(502):44-7.
146. Zakerkish M, Shahbazian HB, Shahbazian H, Latifi SM, Aleali AM. Albuminuria and its correlates in type 2 diabetic patients. Iranian journal of kidney diseases. 2013;7(4):268.
147. Satchell S, Tooke J. What is the mechanism of microalbuminuria in diabetes: a

role for the glomerular endothelium? Diabetologia. 2008;51(5):714-25.
148. De Gaudio A, Adembri C, Grechi S, Novelli G. Microalbuminuria as an early index of impairment of glomerular permeability in postoperative septic patients. Intensive care medicine. 2000;26(9):1364-8.
149. Miller W, Bruns D, Hortin G, Sandberg S, Aakre K, McQueen M, et al, editors. Current data on the determination of urinary albumin excretion. Annales de Biologie Clinique; 2010.
150. Osberg I, Chase HP, Garg SK, DeAndrea A, Harris S, Hamilton R, et al. Effects of storage time and temperature on measurement of small concentrations of albumin in urine. Clinical chemistry. 1990;36(8):1428-30.
151. Brinkman JW, de Zeeuw D, Duker JJ, Gansevoort RT, Kema IP, Hillege HL, et al. Falsely low urinary albumin concentrations after prolonged frozen storage of urine samples. Clinical Chemistry. 2005;51(11):2181-3.
152. Elving L, Bakkeren J, Jansen M, de Kat Angelino C, De Nobel E, Van Munster P. Screening for microalbuminuria in patients with diabetes mellitus: frozen storage of urine samples decreases their albumin content. Clinical chemistry. 1989;35(2):308-10.
153. Heerspink HJL, Brinkman JW, Bakker SJ, Gansevoort RT, de Zeeuw D. Update on microalbuminuria as a biomarker in renal and cardiovascular disease. Current opinion in nephrology and hypertension. 2006;15(6):631-6.
154. Comper WD, Osicka TM, Jerums G. High prevalence of immuno-unreactive intact albumin in urine of diabetic patients. American journal of kidney diseases. 2003;41(2):336-42.
155. Osicka TM, Comper WD. Characterization of immunochemically nonreactive urinary albumin. Clinical chemistry. 2004;50(12):2286-91.
156. Osicka TM, Houlihan CA, Chan JG, Jerums G, Comper WD. Albuminuria in patients with type 1 diabetes is directly linked to changes in the lysosome-mediated degradation of albumin during renal passage. Diabetes. 2000;49(9):1579-84.
157. Schalkwijk CG, Stehouwer CD. Vascular complications in diabetes mellitus: the role of endothelial dysfunction. Clinical science. 2005;109(2):143-59.
158. Weir MR. Microalbuminuria in type 2 diabetics: an important, overlooked cardiovascular risk factor. The Journal of Clinical Hypertension. 2004;6(3):134-43.
159. Seronie-Vivien S, Delanaye P, Pieroni L, Mariat C, Froissart M, Cristol J-P, editors. Cystatin C: point d'étape et perspectives. Annales de Biologie Clinique; 2008: John Libbey Eurotext.
160. Newman DJ. Cystatin c. Annals of clinical biochemistry. 2002;39(2):89-104.
161. Chollet-Dallon E, Stoermann-Chopard C, MARTIN P-Y. Can cystatin C replace creatinine as a marker of glomerular filtration rate: Nephrology. Swiss Medical Journal. 2006;2(55):582-5.
162. Chollet-Dallon E, Stoermann-Chopard C, Martin P. Can cystatin C replace

creatinine as a marker of glomerular filtration rate? Swiss Medical Journal. 2006;55:582.

163. Guyon M. La cystatine C: un nouveau marqueur de la fonction rénale? UHP-Université Henri Poincaré; 2001.

164. Fricker M, Wiesli P, Brändle M, Schwegler B, Schmid C. Impact of thyroid dysfunction on serum cystatin C. Kidney international. 2003;63(5):1944-7.

165. Delanaye P, Chapelle J-P, Gielen J, Krzesinski J-M, Rorive G. The value of cystatin C in the evaluation of renal function. Nephrology. 2003;24(8):457-68.

166. Laterza OF, Price CP, Scott MG. Cystatin C: an improved estimator of glomerular filtration rate? Clinical chemistry. 2002;48(5):699-707.

167. Matsushita K, Van der Velde M, Astor B, Woodward M, Levey A, De Jong P, et al. Chronic Kidney Disease Prognosis Consortium: Association of estimated glomerular filtration rate and albuminuria with all-cause and cardiovascular mortality in general population cohorts: A collaborative meta-analysis. Lancet. 2010;375(9731):2073-81.

168. Inker LA, Schmid CH, Tighiouart H, Eckfeldt JH, Feldman HI, Greene T, et al. Estimating glomerular filtration rate from serum creatinine and cystatin C. New England Journal of Medicine. 2012;367(1):20-9.

169. Stevens LA, Schmid CH, Greene T, Li L, Beck GJ, Joffe MM, et al. Factors other than glomerular filtration rate affect serum cystatin C levels. Kidney international. 2009;75(6):652-60.

170. Wallace A, Price A, Fleischer E, Khoury M, Filler G. Estimation of GFR in patients with cystic fibrosis: a cross-sectional study. Canadian Journal of Kidney Health and Disease. 2020;7:2054358119899312.

171. Mussap M, Dalla Vestra M, Fioretto P, Saller A, Varagnolo M, Nosadini R, et al. Cystatin C is a more sensitive marker than creatinine for the estimation of GFR in type 2 diabetic patients. Kidney Int. 2002;61(4):1453-61. Epub 2002/03/29.

172. Shlipak MG, Sarnak MJ, Katz R, Fried LF, Seliger SL, Newman AB, et al. Cystatin C and the risk of death and cardiovascular events among elderly persons. New England Journal of Medicine. 2005;352(20):2049-60.

173. Lassus J, Harjola V-P. Cystatin C: a step forward in assessing kidney function and cardiovascular risk. Heart failure reviews. 2012;17(2):251-61.

174. Anouar MR, Idmoussa A, El Jahiri Y, Boukhira A, Beraou A, Chellak S. Intérêt du dosage de la bêta-2-microglobuline dans différents milieux biologiques. Revue Francophone des Laboratoires. 2011;2011(436):77-82.

175. Terrier N, Bonardet A, Descomps B, Cristol J, Dupuy A. Determination of beta-2-microglobulin in biological fluids by immunoassay: comparison of RIA, immunohaemiluminescence and immunoturbidimetry. Immunoanalysis & Specialist Biology. 2004;19(4):219-24.

176. Inker LA, Tighiouart H, Coresh J, Foster MC, Anderson AH, Beck GJ, et al. GFR

estimation using β-trace protein and ß2-microglobulin in CKD. American journal of kidney diseases. 2016;67(1):40-8.
177. Filler G, Alvarez-Elías AC, Westreich KD, Huang S-HS, Lindsay RM. Can the new CKD-EPI BTP-B2M formula be applied in children? Pediatric Nephrology. 2016;31(12):2175-7.
178. Yoo C, Yoon DH, Kim S, Huh J, Park CS, Park CJ, et al. Serum beta-2 microglobulin as a prognostic biomarker in patients with mantle cell lymphoma. Hematological oncology. 2016;34(1):22-7.
179. Wakabayashi K, Inokuma S, Matsubara E, Onishi K, Asashima H, Nakachi S, et al. Serum β 2-microglobulin level is a useful indicator of disease activity and hemophagocytic syndrome complication in systemic lupus erythematosus and adult-onset Still's disease. Clinical rheumatology. 2013;32:999-1005.
180. Gluhovschi C, Gluhovschi G, Petrica L, Timar R, Velciov S, Ionita I, et al. Urinary biomarkers in the assessment of early diabetic nephropathy. Journal of diabetes research. 2016;2016.
181. Uwaezuoke SN. The role of novel biomarkers in predicting diabetic nephropathy: a review. International journal of nephrology and renovascular disease. 2017;10:221.
182. Satirapoj B. Tubulointerstitial Biomarkers for Diabetic Nephropathy. J Diabetes Res. 2018;2018:2852398. Epub 2018/03/27.
183. Satirapoj B. Tubulointerstitial biomarkers for diabetic nephropathy. Journal of diabetes research. 2018;2018.
184. Mahfouz MH, Assiri AM, Mukhtar MH. Assessment of neutrophil gelatinase-associated lipocalin (NGAL) and retinol-binding protein 4 (RBP4) in type 2 diabetic patients with nephropathy. Biomarker insights. 2016;11:BMI. S33191.
185. Chou K-M, Lee C-C, Chen C-H, Sun C-Y. Clinical value of NGAL, L-FABP and albuminuria in predicting GFR decline in type 2 diabetes mellitus patients. PLoS One. 2013;8(1):e54863.
186. Papadopoulou-Marketou N, Kanaka-Gantenbein C, Marketos N, Chrousos GP, Papassotiriou I. Biomarkers of diabetic nephropathy: a 2017 update. Critical reviews in clinical laboratory sciences. 2017;54(5):326-42.
187. Khan NU, Lin J, Liu X, Li H, Lu W, Zhong Z, et al. Insights into predicting diabetic nephropathy using urinary biomarkers. Biochimica et Biophysica Acta (BBA)-Proteins and Proteomics. 2020;1868(10):140475.
188. Narita T, Hosoba M, Miura T, Sasaki H, Morii T, Fujita H, et al. Low dose of losartan decreased urinary excretions of IgG, transferrin, and ceruloplasmin without reducing albuminuria in normoalbuminuric type 2 diabetic patients. Hormone and metabolic research. 2008;40(04):292-5.
189. Narita T, Sasaki H, Hosoba M, Miura T, Yoshioka N, Morii T, et al. Parallel increase in urinary excretion rates of immunoglobulin G, ceruloplasmin, transferrin,

and orosomucoid in normoalbuminuric type 2 diabetic patients. Diabetes care. 2004;27(5):1176-81.

190. Tan Y, Yang Y, Zhang Z, Zhang X, Zhang Z, Liu Y. Urinary type IV collagen: a specific indicator of incipient diabetic nephropathy. Chinese medical journal. 2002;115(03):389- 94.

191. Banu N, Hara H, Okamura M, Egusa G, Yamakido M. Urinary excretion of type IV collagen and laminin in the evaluation of nephropathy in NIDDM: comparison with urinary albumin and markers of tubular dysfunction and/or damage. Diabetes Research and Clinical Practice. 1995;29(1):57-67.

192. Haiyashi Y, Makino H, Ota Z. Serum and urinary concentrations of type IV collagen and laminin as a marker of microangiopathy in diabetes. Diabetic medicine. 1992;9(4):366-70.

193. Torffvit O. Urinary sulphated glycosaminoglycans and Tamm-Horsfall protein in type 1 diabetic patients. Scandinavian journal of urology and nephrology. 1999;33(5):328- 32.

194. Coca SG, Nadkarni GN, Huang Y, Moledina DG, Rao V, Zhang J, et al. Plasma Biomarkers and Kidney Function Decline in Early and Established Diabetic Kidney Disease. J Am Soc Nephrol. 2017;28(9):2786-93. Epub 2017/05/10.

195. Perlman AS, Chevalier JM, Wilkinson P, Liu H, Parker T, Levine DM, et al. Serum inflammatory and immune mediators are elevated in early stage diabetic nephropathy. Annals of Clinical & Laboratory Science. 2015;45(3):256-63.

196. Uwaezuoke SN. The role of novel biomarkers in predicting diabetic nephropathy: a review. International journal of nephrology and renovascular disease. 2017:221-31.

197. Wu LL, Chiou C-C, Chang P-Y, Wu JT. Urinary 8-OHdG: a marker of oxidative stress to DNA and a risk factor for cancer, atherosclerosis and diabetics. Clinica chimica acta. 2004;339(1-2):1-9.

198. Li X, Lu L, Hou W, Huang T, Chen X, Qi J, et al. Epigenetics in the pathogenesis of diabetic nephropathy. Acta Biochimica et Biophysica Sinica. 2022;54(2):1-10.

199. Kato M, Natarajan R. Diabetic nephropathy-emerging epigenetic mechanisms. Nature Reviews Nephrology. 2014;10(9):517-30.

200. Musante L, Tataruch DE, Holthofer H. Use and isolation of urinary exosomes as biomarkers for diabetic nephropathy. Frontiers in endocrinology. 2014;5:149.

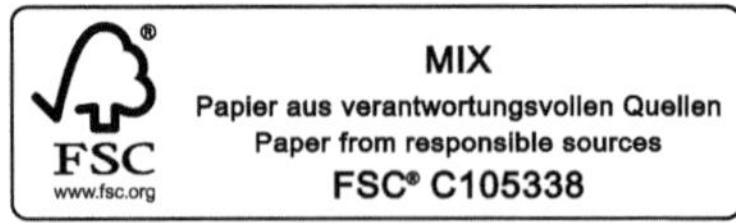

Printed by Books on Demand GmbH, Norderstedt / Germany